Intentionally Infecting Humans

Intentionally Infecting Humans

Is It Ethical?

SEEMA K. SHAH

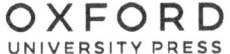

OXFORD
UNIVERSITY PRESS

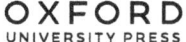

OXFORD
UNIVERSITY PRESS

Oxford University Press is a department of the University of Oxford.
It furthers the University's objective of excellence in research, scholarship,
and education by publishing worldwide. Oxford is a registered trade mark of
Oxford University Press in the UK and in certain other countries.

Published in the United States of America by Oxford University Press
198 Madison Avenue, New York, NY 10016, United States of America.

CIP data is on file at the Library of Congress

ISBN 9780197667897

DOI: 10.1093/9780197667927.001.0001

Printed by Integrated Books International, United States of America

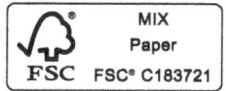

The manufacturer's authorized representative in the EU for product safety is
Oxford University Press España S.A. of Parque Empresarial San Fernando de Henares,
Avenida de Castilla, 2 – 28830 Madrid (www.oup.es/en or product.safety@oup.com).
OUP España S.A. also acts as importer into Spain of products made by the manufacturer.

For Frank Miller and Christine Grady, who launched this conversation about the ethics of controlled human infection research and included me in it.

Contents

Preface

By the turn of the twentieth century, yellow fever had caused multiple epidemics and killed more than 100,000 people in the United States alone (Patterson, 1992). Yet scientists did not understand what caused the deadly disease to spread. To that end, Dr. Walter Reed was appointed to lead a special commission to study yellow fever (Lederer, 2008). Reed planned to investigate two competing theories about how yellow fever could be transmitted. One theory was that yellow fever was spread through contact with the bodily fluids of people who were sick; the alternative was that mosquitoes transmitted the disease from person to person. To settle this debate, Walter Reed's research team set up a site in Cuba and ran several risky experiments (Reed, 1902). These experiments required doing something that seems contrary to the central purpose of medicine—they were trying to make healthy people sick.

The most famous of these experiments involved randomly assigning volunteers to stay in one of two uninviting conditions. One hut was filled with bedsheets and surfaces covered in fluids that came from yellow fever patients. Others were assigned to stay in a tent filled with mosquitos that had just fed on yellow fever patients. When the volunteers became sick from mosquitos but not from bodily fluids, the experiment definitively settled the question of how yellow fever was transmitted. This discovery led to near elimination of yellow fever in countries that could rid themselves of mosquitoes that carried it and saved countless lives—a tremendous public health achievement (Sutter, 2016).

At that time in history, research ethics was in its infancy. Indeed, Walter Reed's experiment was followed by decades of studies involving intentional infection that were ethically problematic or even "ethically impossible" (Presidential Commission for the Study of Bioethical Issues, 2011). Yet Walter Reed's team had an unusual sensitivity to the ethics of their research. Although the level of risk that volunteers undertook was much higher than what would likely pass muster with an ethics review board today, volunteers were given an early contract that was essentially an informed consent document—which was not standard practice at the time. The researchers paid participants in gold and promised to pay additional funds to the relatives of anyone who died in the study (Lederer, 2008). In this respect in particular, the ethics of this study were remarkably advanced. Despite several bioethics commissions recommending that research participants receive compensation if they are injured by research, compensation for research-related injury is still not required in the United States today (Pike, 2014). These yellow fever experiments provide an early example that demonstrates both the potential power and ethical complexity of exposing people to pathogens for science—not to mention the way that this unusual type of research can spur innovation in ethics, which is a central theme of this book.

I first became interested in controlled human infection (CHI) research in 2014, when I was at the Department of Bioethics at the National Institutes of Health, serving as a liaison to the National Institute of Allergy and Infectious Diseases (NIAID). In that role, I was asked to help moderate a debate at NIAID on whether CHI research could be ethically acceptable. The leaders of the two divisions within NIAID took opposing positions on the topic, and I presented an ethical analysis that I intended to provide a more balanced view. At the time, I was fortunate to receive advice from the first two ethicists who had written a manuscript focused on the ethics of CHI research—Frank Miller and Christine Grady—and I drew heavily on their seminal work. What I did not realize at the time, though, was how much more work needed to be done. In 2016, after I had moved to another institution, I was asked to chair a National Institutes of Health (NIH) panel on ethical considerations for CHI research with Zika virus, which was then emerging. I was reluctant to take on this role, recognizing how controversial the topic was at the time, but felt confident that we could rely on the existing ethical analyses in the literature and simply apply it to the case of CHI research with Zika virus. As illustrated in Chapter 5, I could not have been more wrong. This book is the product of more than a decade of work to address the challenging and sometimes unresolved ethical questions raised by CHI research.

Before providing an overview of what this book sets out to accomplish to add clarity to the ethics of CHI research, however, I will briefly address terminology, which is a surprisingly complicated issue.

Briefly Defining the Terms

In CHI research, researchers intentionally expose small numbers of participants to pathogens to gain scientific insights. CHI research is a particularly powerful way to learn about interactions between diseases and hosts and/or test experimental vaccines or treatments (Roestenberg et al., 2018). CHI research is known by different names, including *human challenge studies*, *trials*, or *models* and *voluntary infection studies*. In fact, the Wellcome Trust commissioned a report focused exclusively on the terminology used for these studies (Marsh, 2018).

In this book, I use the term "controlled human infection (CHI)" research as an umbrella term that covers both CHI models and CHI studies. Developing a CHI model is the first step in the process; only once a CHI model has been shown to be safe and reliable can it be used in CHI studies to test interventions like vaccines and treatments. I further explain the difference between CHI models and studies in Chapter 3, when it becomes important for understanding what makes this research unique and how this research can be conducted ethically—for example, it will help clarify when extra oversight is needed. While I will use this approach to terminology in most of the book, the only exception is when I discuss historical examples of studies, in Chapter 1 and throughout the book, that were conducted before the modern oversight system for research was developed. In those instances, I will use the terminology used at the time the studies were conducted: "human challenge trials."

Why Analyze the Ethics of Intentionally Infecting Humans?

CHI research has been integral to ground-breaking scientific achievements. In addition to the discovery that yellow fever was transmitted by mosquitoes, discussed at the start of the introduction and in greater depth in Chapter 1, a smallpox challenge conducted by Edward Jenner proved the concept of vaccinology (Riedel, 2005). With the advent of increased ethical safeguards for research in the 1980s, CHI studies have been powerful tools for accelerating the development of new treatments and vaccines. To date, more than 15,000 people have participated in human challenge studies for at least 30 pathogen models (Abo et al., 2023). A traveler's cholera vaccine and a typhoid vaccine were recently approved, relying heavily on data from CHI research. The use of CHI studies is a standard part of the testing of any new interventions for malaria, including a recently approved malaria vaccine (Roestenberg et al., 2018). Yet the exciting scientific promise of these studies can be tempered by their potential for ethical abuses and controversy. For example, to prove the concept of vaccination, Jenner enlisted his gardener's 8-year-old son without clearly obtaining consent and exposed him to cowpox and then smallpox (Riedel, 2005).

Greater ethical clarity is also sorely needed regarding how to use CHI research ethically to address emerging infectious disease threats. As mentioned above, in 2017, I was invited to chair an expert panel of ethicists, clinicians, and researchers that was convened by the National Institute of Allergy and Infectious Diseases to determine whether it was ethical to develop a CHI model with Zika virus. Our panel recommended pausing the proposed CHI research involving Zika virus based on two ethical issues we could not resolve at the time: the unclear value of the research and concerns about risk to third parties outside of the study who could not give their consent (Shah et al., 2018). The panel struggled with this decision, as discussed in Chapter 5. Some thought too little was known about the virus to conduct such studies ethically, especially in terms of how to protect members of the public from being infected by volunteers participating in the study. On the other hand, since Zika virus was spreading rapidly, others felt that any tool should be used to prevent the peril involved, including deliberately infecting people with Zika virus in research. In fact, in an article published in the *New York Times*, our recommendation to pause the study was described as having "slammed the door on progress" (Baumgaertner, 2018). Controversy involving the Zika CHI model persisted for a time, but, as more evidence about transmission of Zika virus emerged and the ethical issues could be addressed, the Zika CHI model was allowed to proceed (Vannice et al., 2019). Before it could be resumed, however, the nascent global debate over CHI research was taken to another level.

During the COVID-19 pandemic, research involving deliberate human infection with a pathogen was hotly debated as a way to respond to the spread of this new disease that had stopped the world in its tracks (Eyal et al., 2020; Kahn et al., 2020; McPartlin et al., 2020). The potential use of CHI research to accelerate the development of a vaccine against the novel coronavirus captured the public's imagination, not to mention the attention of ethicists. After decades of the ethics of CHI research being a niche topic, in 2020, there was an explosion of papers on the subject, with more than 100 ethics papers written in the first year of the pandemic—more than ever before or since (Katzer et al., 2023).

In addition to the unprecedented scholarly attention to CHI research, a new organization called "1Day Sooner" ran such a successful advocacy campaign for CHI research that they were vaulted into the public consciousness. 1Day Sooner established a registry that ultimately included more than 38,000 willing volunteers and drummed up media interest in the topic, in addition to generating several open letters that were signed by prominent academics and other figures (1Day Sooner, 2020). Their efforts interested members of Congress, who asked Dr. Anthony Fauci to respond about why the NIH was not conducting these studies. Despite the fact that CHI research with COVID-19 has now been conducted in the United Kingdom, with more research being planned (Rapeport et al., 2021), this research was not done in the United States and other countries in part due to ethical concerns (Gupta et al., 2020). The sharp divides that arose during the COVID-19 pandemic are less surprising when viewed in context, however. Ethical concerns about CHI research have persisted throughout its long, complex history (Bambery et al., 2016) and are worthy of further examination.

Key Contributions

This book seeks to make two key contributions. The first is to advance the debate about CHI research by focusing attention on when it requires additional ethical scrutiny. Scholars have typically treated CHI research in one of two ways: either it is seen as raising unprecedented ethical questions that always require extra scrutiny, or it has been considered no different from other types of research. I will demonstrate that CHI research is not monolithic and falls on a wide spectrum of value, risk, and uncertainty. I will further show that CHI research has surprising similarities to other types of research but will argue that CHI research is ethically distinct because it can raise several difficult, unresolved ethical issues at the same time. When CHI research raises this unusual set of unresolved ethical issues, extra scrutiny can be helpful to ensure the research is conducted ethically, if it is justifiable to conduct it at all.

Importantly, I will make an ethical distinction between CHI models and studies. As will be explained later, a CHI model for how to infect people reliably and safely is just the first step in the process. Creating a new CHI model therefore involves making several decisions that will affect any studies that will be done with the model in the future. I will argue in Chapter 4 that, as a general rule, CHI models should have extra scrutiny and specialized review, whereas CHI studies can go through standard review processes and be evaluated by an Institutional Review Board or Research Ethics Committee. In that chapter, I also provide a framework to help guide the ethical conduct of CHI research. Use of this framework will help make clear when CHI research should be treated the same as other types of research and when it requires specialized review to rigorously evaluate the difficult and unresolved issues this type of research can raise. My goal is to take the temperature down for certain types of CHI research and increase ethical caution surrounding others.

This framework will also help clarify how CHI research should proceed when moving into new populations. For example, as India contemplates conducting its first CHI research, for example, beginning with established CHI studies that pose lower risk and less uncertainty than new models will help build the capacity and public trust needed to support more of this research in the future.

A second contribution is to clarify how CHI research can be used ethically and effectively. CHI research suffers from an abundance of hype and a lack of clarity about how and why it can be valuable for society in the first place. Indeed, in considering whether to use CHI research during the COVID-19 pandemic, many focused on whether CHI studies should play a primary role as the final phase of vaccine testing or none at all. The other ways that CHI research can be and has been useful—for example, by yielding fundamental insights about diseases or playing supporting roles in vaccine and treatment development—received less attention. I will argue that CHI research should generally be seen as a long-term investment in accelerating the development of new vaccines and treatments rather than a last-minute shortcut. In Chapter 5, I show how CHI research during the COVID-19 pandemic was ethically problematic precisely because it was sold as a "quick fix" to make vaccines available at least one day sooner. Using a longer-term lens to evaluate CHI research can help to avoid such mistakes in the future.

Finally, it is also worth noting that, although this book is written primarily for an academic audience, I have attempted to write it in a way that will be accessible to members of the public and policymakers, to illuminate the unique role that these studies can and, most importantly, should play. In recognition of the many important perspectives on CHI research, each chapter begins with a quote from someone who has volunteered to participate in a CHI model or study, drawn from the largest set of qualitative data from potential volunteers for challenge studies, which was gathered through a collaboration with the organization 1Day Sooner.

Overview

This book proceeds in three parts. First, I set the stage for an analysis of CHI research. Next, I provide an ethical framework to guide the evaluation of CHI research. Finally, I look ahead to implications of this analysis for future studies in other contexts, with new populations, or in future pandemics. I close by considering the implications of this analysis more broadly.

Part I

I begin by providing a historical overview of CHI research in Chapter 1. There have been several exploitative and unethical studies involving CHI research, including studies that exposed people to high risks with limited chances of social or personal benefit, and research in which participants were never asked for their consent. This history of ethically questionable research colors the conduct of CHI research to this day. This history also reveals that CHI research usually provides value by demonstrating why some people are better protected from disease than others, how transmission of infections occurs, and how correlates of protection can be used as proxy measures to enable larger clinical trials to obtain faster results. There are few examples of CHI research being used to provide the primary data for approval of vaccines or treatments, which was the initial reason CHI research received so much attention during the COVID-19 pandemic. Ultimately, Chapter 1 provides historical grounding that can explain why it is so critical for CHI research to be conducted to the highest scientific and ethical standards to not repeat the mistakes of the past and to support the public trust that CHI research needs to be successful.

In Chapter 2, I address what scholars have referred to as a "yuck factor" associated with these studies. In other words, people often intuitively react to the idea of CHI research as inherently unethical. Although scholars have argued that CHI research is not ethically distinct except insofar as the work might threaten public trust in research, I take this opportunity to analyze the question in greater depth and argue to the contrary. I examine research behind the "yuck" factor to better understand why people might react to CHI research in this way, including considering whether different types of challenge studies can raise higher "yuck" reactions than others. Finally, I explain why we should take the "yuck" factor seriously, even though it does not necessarily track moral truths, and I suggest a way to address it directly.

In Chapter 3, I build on this analysis to dive into a key philosophical issue that has not received the treatment it deserves: asking whether CHI research is ethically unique. The aim of this chapter will be to isolate whether there are objective moral reasons to treat CHI research differently from other types of research or other activities, or whether misfiring intuitions and subjective judgments make CHI research feel ethically distinct. I ultimately argue that CHI research is unusual because of the set of complex and/or unresolved ethical issues it raises, particularly when embarking on research that intentionally exposes humans to a pathogen for the first time, that can merit extra ethical scrutiny.

Part II

In the second part of the book, I provide an ethical framework to guide the evaluation of CHI research that will help clarify when CHI research can go through standard review processes and when additional scrutiny may be needed. In Chapter 4, I lay out the ethical frameworks contained in existing World Health Organization (WHO) guidance as well as an ethical framework I have previously developed with a multidisciplinary, international group to articulate criteria for the use of challenge studies. I first situate the framework within current ethics literature and guidance documents for CHI research to provide a full account of the range of views on CHI research. I then lay out the framework and show how using the framework with the distinction between CHI models and studies in mind can help balance risk and reward in the use of CHI research as well as illuminate red lines that should not be crossed.

I then apply this framework to CHI research on emerging infectious diseases in Chapter 5, given the high level of uncertainty entailed in infecting people with a disease that is poorly understood. I examine examples of a CHI model for Zika virus and CHI research conducted in the United Kingdom during the COVID-19 pandemic and draw out lessons for the use of CHI research in pandemic preparedness. I argue that treating CHI research as a quick fix is generally ethically suspect and will not provide a good return on investment. To help avoid such mistakes in the future, CHI research should be considered just one part of a longer-term research strategy to develop vaccines and treatments.

Part III

In the final part of the book, I look ahead to how CHI research should be used in the future and what it can teach us about the ethics of research in general before tying everything together in the final chapter. In Chapter 6, I consider the expansion of CHI research into new populations, such as the use of CHI research in low- and middle-income countries. CHI research is increasingly being used in low- and middle-income countries (e.g., Kenya, Zambia, and Vietnam) to address diseases that have higher burdens in these countries (Jamrozik & Selgelid, 2020b). Some scholars have even argued there is an "ethical imperative" to conduct CHI research in low- and middle-income countries, provided appropriate safeguards are in place, if it can help accelerate access to treatments and vaccines to address the disproportionate disease burdens shouldered by these countries (Jamrozik & Selgelid, 2020a). CHI research in low- and middle-income countries can also raise concerns about exploitation and global justice, particularly in light of a movement to decolonize global health (Abimbola & Pai, 2020), and these concerns may merit additional attention. I also consider the expansion of CHI research into different populations that may be at higher risks, such as immunocompromised people, children, and pregnant people. Most ethical frameworks and guidance documents have counseled against inclusion of these groups or merely suggested it should be considered; I attempt to clarify how it can be ethical to include these groups in certain categories of CHI research but important to exclude them from others.

Next, I consider the broader implications of this analysis for CHI research in particular and human subjects research in general in Chapter 7. Because CHI research raises a set of issues that are unresolved in research ethics, sustained analysis should allow for progress in these important areas. The research ethics literature has not resolved questions as wide-ranging as how to measure the social value of research, what limits can be placed on the right to withdraw, how to address third-party risks, and how to consider the need for public trust in research when evaluating particular studies. For example, the advocacy by research participants during the COVID-19 pandemic reveals a need to elevate the act of participating in research.

Research participants have typically received public attention when they have been harmed or exploited in research. Consider, for example, James Phipps, the 8-year-old child famous for having been exposed to smallpox by Edward Jenner, or Jesse Gelsinger, who died in a gene therapy trial that was subject to substantial ethical criticism. The discussion of CHI research and the prominence of the advocacy organization 1DaySooner during the COVID-19 pandemic present an opportunity to decrease the stigma associated with research participation and promote greater societal respect for research participants and their contributions to scientific advances (Kraft et al., 2023).

The final chapter gathers the lessons learned throughout the book to provide a cohesive, higher-level overview of the ethics of intentionally infecting humans in research.

Conclusion

CHI research puts into stark relief the question of when it is ethically acceptable to expose some people to risk for the benefit of others. My hope is that diving into the ethics of this fascinating and controversial research method can help illuminate the path to the ethical use of CHI research in the future and advance the field of research ethics along the way.

Acknowledgments

I began writing this book in 2020 and have had much help along the way. First, my former colleagues from the National Institutes of Health (NIH) have contributed a great deal to this work. I am very grateful to Frank Miller for reviewing Chapters 1–5, identifying gaps, asking many astute questions, and bolstering my confidence when I needed it most. I am deeply thankful to Christine Grady, who first suggested that I participate in a debate over the ethics of controlled human infection (CHI) research during a retreat at the National Institute of Allergy and Infectious Diseases and who has long elevated me to opportunities I would never have imagined for myself. My former mentor, David Wendler, reviewed Chapter 2 of this book and provided helpful feedback on the proposal and title with his characteristic generosity, for which I am very grateful. I thank Zeke Emanuel for suggesting the title and pushing me to be bolder. Annette Rid has been one of my closest collaborators on this work on the ethics of CHI research over several years; she has helped me work through so many of these ideas in their more nascent forms, including the distinction between CHI models and studies and the ethical framework—often over dishes and late at night. I am also grateful for the many articles she sent me to enrich this manuscript and for her friendship, which made doing this work so much more enjoyable.

I thank the incredibly gracious Bob Eisinger for supporting my leadership on an NIH panel that galvanized my thinking in this area and for keeping me abreast of relevant literature and scientific developments that I drew on to write this book. I am also grateful to the colleagues who served with me on that panel—and to Holly Lynch and Jonathan Kimmelman in particular—for helping advance my thinking on the ethics of CHI research in many ways.

Lucy Randall was a dream editor who gave me the space and freedom to write the best book I could and supported my efforts to fund the time to write it. She also leads a stellar editorial and production team, including Jodie Keefe, and identified anonymous reviewers who were knowledgeable, thoughtful, encouraging, and eminently fair. Their suggestions have strengthened this book immensely. I also thank the design team for their patience and thoughtful approach to the cover art.

I am deeply grateful to the Sloan Foundation for their support of my writing time on this project and for research assistance, along with the Greenwall Foundation and Brocher Foundation for funding the work that led to this project.

I would like to thank the participants at the Charm City Colloquium for their suggestions on Chapter 4. Debra Mathews, Safura Abdool Karim, and Leslie Wolf had especially valuable insights. I am also grateful to Roli Mathur, Anu Rose, Reidar Lie, Robert Steel, and other participants of the Indo-US workshop who helped me think through the contributions of CHI research for India and other low- and middle-income countries in Chapter 6. Vivian David Jacob's insights were invaluable and helped me identify the reasons that low- and middle-income countries could benefit from CHI research. He also read carefully through the entire book, suggesting missing literature, finding factual errors, and identifying places where I had not yet accomplished what I said I would do, for which I am very grateful.

I appreciate my colleagues at Northwestern and Lurie Children's Hospital who have supported this effort in various ways. Sidney Halpern's review of Chapter 1 was meticulous; her suggestions made the brief historical account of CHIs more accurate and factually grounded. I am indebted to Barbara Deal, not only for being our only source of childcare in the first few months of the COVID-19 pandemic, but also for advising me on how to go about writing a book in an academic medical center. Michelle Macy similarly supported me in carving out the space to write while fulfilling my other duties. I am tremendously grateful to Matt Davis, whose mentorship was essential for keeping me on the path to writing this book, and who provided valuable suggestions on the introduction and Chapters 1 and 2.

I was very fortunate to work with students and research staff who contributed a great deal of time and effort to improving the book. Rick Weinmeyer helped with references, proofreading, and identifying where my writing could be tightened and strengthened. Olivia Orr was always willing to help and pitched in several times throughout the process, particularly with proofreading, endnotes, and drafting the index. It was a genuine pleasure to collaborate with Jeffrey Poomkudy to work through how virtue theory provides insights about CHI studies, which also helped me refine my view of what makes CHI research unique. Ava Jurden and Akram Ibrahim kept my other projects humming while I spent time on this one; Ava also helped bring my vision for the cover to life. Laniya Lucas brought endless cheerfulness, warmth, and reminders to prioritize this project when so many other things required attention. I am incredibly thankful to these colleagues for their support.

I am very thankful to the CHI researchers who helped me understand this research method—Ricardo Palacios, Meta Roestenberg, Sean Murphy, Tom Richie, Melissa Kapulu, and Tom Darton in particular deserve special mention. Tom Darton's comments on Chapter 5 were incredibly helpful; I also appreciate his willingness to talk through the distinction between models and studies as I was still working it out.

Steven Chao's comments on the first few chapters also helped me see how to make the book more useful to those who are not immersed in ethics or CHI research; I am so fortunate to have him as a friend. I would be remiss if I did not mention Alan Wertheimer, without whose mentorship I would not have been in a position to write this manuscript. I hope this book does his investment in me justice.

There are so many more people to thank for their support— including my wonderful in-laws, my peer mentors and friends, and the members of my communities. Though I lack the space to name them all, I am so grateful for the countless ways they have sustained me in this work.

Finally, I thank my family for putting up with me throughout this process, and particularly so on those vacation mornings when I parked myself in front of a laptop and was no fun at all. This book simply would not have happened without my sister Nisha, who was on call at all hours for technical support, pep talks, amateur therapy sessions, and consulting on strategic decisions. I thank my mom for her endless support and for always reminding me to write a book before it was too late, and my dad for his confidence in me and for proofreading multiple chapters. I am grateful to my spouse Mahesh for so many things, including but not limited to the following: watching the girls in foreign countries while I attended meetings and developed key insights for this book, making me laugh during the lowest points of the writing process, and being a wonderful collaborator on this twist in our adventure. Finally, Salila and Shivani: thank you for always providing your loving and honest feedback, keeping me humble, and making it all worthwhile; I cannot wait to make up for lost time now that this book is finally written.

1

A Historical Overview of Challenge Studies

Promise and Peril

> I believe people should be allowed to make calculated
> risks that benefit others. We do this in many other areas of
> life, but their [sic] is such a complicated and ugly history
> with medicine that we have completely moved away from
> this model.
> —Prospective volunteer for COVID-19 CHI research

In controlled human infection (CHI) research, researchers deliberately expose volunteers to pathogens to learn more about diseases or efficiently test new interventions. CHI research has been conducted for more than 200 years; it is commonly referred to by other names, including "challenge studies"—a term that was once the standard (Roestenberg et al., 2018). While I will generally use the term "CHI research" to refer to present-day or potential research, I will follow the convention of describing historical examples as "challenge studies," in line with how they were described when they were conducted. In fact, modern researchers may have turned to new terminology to communicate that their work is different from infamous challenge studies in the past.

Many historical challenge studies raised serious ethical concerns; in fact, some have been described as "ethically impossible" (Presidential Commission for the Study of Bioethical Issues, 2011). Revisiting this history simultaneously reveals both the promise and peril of this research method. These historical challenge studies illustrate different types of ethical breaches and help identify lines that should not be crossed in this type of research. While challenge

Intentionally Infecting Humans. Seema K. Shah, Oxford University Press. © Seema K. Shah 2026.
DOI: 10.1093/9780197667927.003.0001

studies were responsible for tremendous scientific breakthroughs, including proving the concept of vaccination and identifying that mosquitoes transmit yellow fever, even some of the most celebrated scientific achievements have entailed exploitation of participants from marginalized groups who were unable to protect themselves.

In this chapter, I trace the history of challenge studies to diagnose ethical concerns and dangers associated with this research method. My goal is not to conduct an exhaustive review of the historical use of this method but rather to examine several important cases of historical challenge studies to understand the potential scientific contributions and the ethical lapses in the conduct of this research. I argue that the historical abuses of the past continue to cast a shadow on modern-day CHI research and demonstrate why some groups continue to lack trust in CHI research today, making it critical for modern-day CHI research to be conducted in line with rigorous scientific and ethical standards.

Origins of Intentional Human Infection

People have been deliberately exposing themselves and others to pathogens for a long time. To protect against smallpox, some practiced *variolation*, which involved inserting pus from smallpox patients into the skin of healthy patients to train their immune systems with a mild infection that would ultimately generate protection from future exposures. While variolation posed a 2–3% risk of death, the alternative was worse. The mortality rate from smallpox was between 20% and 60% in adults (Riedel, 2005). Variolation was used in Asia and Africa for hundreds of years; it was documented as occurring in China as early as 1695 (Plotkin & Plotkin, 2018). In the 1700s, variolation came to Europe when a British ambassador's wife, Lady Mary Wortley Montague, took up the cause. Lady Montague had previously been disfigured after a bout of smallpox, and she lost her brother to the disease. She encountered variolation in Istanbul, noting, "Every year, thousands undergo this operation, and the French ambassador says pleasantly that they take the smallpox here by way of diversion as they do the waters in other countries" (National Library of Medicine, 2011). In the early 1700s, a physician named Charles Maitland was permitted by the royal family to test variation in people incarcerated at Newgate Prison. The participants in this experiment were promised a pardon if they followed through with it. In what was perhaps the earliest challenge study, these participants went through variation and were then exposed to people with smallpox; no one was infected with smallpox, and they all survived. Dr. Maitland repeated his experiment in children who had been orphaned (another captive population) (Lederer, 2014). After members of the British royal family underwent variation in 1722, it became more widely accepted.

Variation took hold slightly later in North America. During a smallpox outbreak in Boston (Pasteur, 1881), an enslaved man from Africa called Onesimus explained the practice to Cotton Mather, who then encouraged members of his community to adopt variation. Cotton Mather was a Puritan priest, infamous for his pivotal role in the Salem Witch Trials; Mather's congregation had purchased Onesimus for him (Najera, 2020). In the late 1700s, variation took a step closer to vaccination when used by a cattle breeder named Benjamin Jesty. Recognizing that dairymaids were protected from smallpox after having had the milder disease known as cowpox, Jesty deliberately exposed himself and his family to cowpox—but not smallpox (Baxby, 1985). This was not an example of research, as Jesty acted to protect his own family and did not design and test a method that could be used by others.

The first clear example of a challenge study occurred in 1796, when a famous series of challenge studies became a proof of concept for vaccination. Edward Jenner drew upon practices of variation to conduct several experiments inoculating adults and children (including infants) with cowpox, sometimes followed by exposure to smallpox. To more "accurately observe the progress of infection," he infected his gardener's son, James Phipps, who was 8 years old at the time. This was the seventeenth case listed in a report Jenner prepared for the King of England. Jenner himself had been inoculated with smallpox as a child. Jenner extracted fluid from cowpox vesicles on the hand of a milkmaid named Sarah Nelmes (Jenner, 1802) and then deliberately exposed Phipps to cowpox. Jenner monitored the mild symptoms of that disease to ensure Phipps had been infected with it and then inoculated Phipps with smallpox 6 weeks later. When Phipps stayed healthy, Jenner concluded that Phipps was protected from infection with smallpox based on his prior exposure to cowpox (Baxby, 1985). Jenner called this procedure "vaccination," after the Latin word for a "cow" (*vacca*).

While the scientific impact of this work led to the eradication of smallpox—an achievement beyond dispute—the ethics remain questionable. It is unclear, but seems unlikely, that Phipps gave his assent or that his parents understood what was involved and gave their permission for his involvement in this experiment. Although this challenge study fell far short of modern standards for informed consent, some have attempted to identify an ethical justification by pointing out that variolation with smallpox was common at the time, making the research consistent with standard practices (Davies, 2007). Indeed, challenge studies using Jenner's methodology and also using children as participants were conducted in London, Paris, Vienna, and Boston (Lederer, 2008). Jenner himself repeated this experiment on other impoverished children and adults, however, raising concerns that his participants were selected due to their vulnerability. Additionally, Jenner was not entirely certain what other pathogens might have been in the substances he used to inoculate others. Indeed, recent research suggests that the smallpox vaccine may have been derived from horsepox (Schrick et al., 2017).

Jenner's approach was common among challenge studies conducted at this time. Researchers subjected people to experiments that left lingering questions about their scientific validity, involved high risks, and exposed infants and children to harm. In the 1800s, for example, European investigators conducted experiments that involved extracting infectious material from patients with sexually transmitted infections, such as gonorrhea and syphilis, and injecting it into infants and young children (Jamrozik & Selgelid, 2020). The discovery and adoption of germ theory was a major advance for research involving intentional infection. Germ theory was proposed by Louis Pasteur in the late 1800s (Pasteur, 1881) and was the subject of lively debate before it began to have sway among the scientific and medical communities (Tomes, 1997). Having an understanding of what caused disease laid a foundation for scientists to conduct research that involved inducing diseases by exposing people to pathogens.

One remarkable example demonstrates how challenge studies can lead to ethical innovation; yet subsequent developments further show how quickly progress can be reversed. In the late 1800s, German scientists such as Albert Neisser conducted research in which they gave sex workers and orphaned children an experimental vaccine against syphilis and then exposed them to syphilis without their consent. These experiments had received advance approval from a parliamentary commission. When these experiments became widely known, there was so much public disapproval that the government produced what was likely the first research ethics directive in the world. This directive emphasized the need to explain potential risks, obtain informed consent, and protect groups who were considered "vulnerable." After another scandal involving an experimental tuberculosis vaccine that caused the deaths of 75 children, the German government developed research ethics regulations in 1931. These regulations codified the protections listed in the first directive and also specifically required additional caution for infection with pathogens, such as in challenge trials. The regulations emphasized the need to make sure deliberate infection was safe and likely to provide the participants with benefits that could not otherwise be attained (Cohen Jr., 2010). Notwithstanding the ethical advancement represented by these early regulations, some of the most horrific challenge studies to date that were conducted in Nazi Germany just a few years after they were passed, as discussed further below.

Returning to the late 1800s, several noteworthy early challenge studies focused on yellow fever. Yellow fever is a flavivirus, like West Nile and Zika viruses, that was responsible for frequent global epidemics in the 1800s and killed 15–50% of patients infected with it. The name "yellow fever" was based on the liver damage it often caused, which could result in jaundice (yellowing of the skin due to high bilirubin levels). In the United States, some postulate that publicity about common yellow fever outbreaks in the Southern states may even have influenced the perception of the South as a poorer, less advanced part of the country (Patterson, 1992). Initially, the theory that yellow fever was caused by a germ of some sort was the dominant view, and it motivated methods of disease control that later proved to be ineffectual, such as the use of powerful disinfectants on ships and their goods after they came into port (Warner, 1985).

During the end of the nineteenth century, researchers raced to uncover the cause of this deadly disease, and challenge studies were used in ways that were sometimes troubling but occasionally brilliant. Domingos Freire was a scientist and proponent of the theory that a microbe he had found in fluids taken from yellow fever patients was the cause of the disease. In the 1880s, Freire created what he believed was a live attenuated vaccine for yellow fever and injected it into hundreds of people in Brazil. His research was later harshly criticized and was unable to be replicated. In 1897, the researcher Giuseppe Sanarelli claimed to have identified a bacterium that caused yellow fever and used it to conduct a poorly conceived challenge study. Sanarelli injected this bacterium into four patients at a hospital in Bolivia, three of whom died after exhibiting symptoms of what he characterized as yellow fever. Researchers who sought to recover Sanarelli's bacteria from yellow fever patients could not find it, however. His results were ultimately discredited when researchers realized that what he identified was likely a form of cholera that causes classical swine fever (or, as it was referred to at the time, "hog cholera") (Reed & Carroll, 1900).

Sanarelli faced criticism for his ethical lapses (Sternberg, 1898). As the prominent physician Arthur Leffingwell wrote, "It is absurd to fancy that the subjects of these experiments knew what was done, when for the relief of some trifling ailment they submitted to the prick of a needle, and were devoted to death.... I have no language at command sufficiently strong to phrase my opinion of a man who, in the garb of a physician, could be guilty of such a crime" (Leffingwell, 1899). Leffingwell was outraged by the fact that Sanarelli had conducted his experiments on the vulnerable and marginalized. A more succinct condemnation came from the notable physician William Osler, who argued that "To deliberately inject a poison of known high degree of virulency into a human being, unless you obtain that man's sanction, is not ridiculous, it is criminal" (Association of American Physicians, 1898).

With several promising candidates for yellow fever eliminated, a new approach was needed. A physician from Cuba named Carlos Finlay had an alternative theory that mosquitoes transmitted yellow fever. Finlay's claim needed proof, however. Enter US Army physician Walter Reed, who was put in charge of the US Yellow Fever Commission. In 1900, the Commission conducted experiments in Cuba to determine how yellow fever was transmitted (Lederer, 2008). In the earliest experiments, individuals were directly inoculated with yellow fever. Later, participants were randomly assigned to one of two conditions, each designed to infect people with yellow fever in different ways. The participants in the study were all described as immigrants to Cuba who lacked immunity to yellow fever (Reed, 1902). Some of them were recent immigrants from Spain, while others were members of the US military (Smith, 2019).

In the first arm of this study, the researchers built a small frame house with only one room that was 14 × 20 feet in size and had minimal circulation. The building had wire screens on the windows and doors to ensure no mosquitoes could enter from outside, including a vestibule with a second wire-screened door after initial entry. The researchers prepared three large boxes with linens (e.g., sheets, pillowcases, and blankets) that were "soiled with a liberal quantity of black vomit, urine, and fecal matter" (Reed, 1902). The volunteers who slept in this hut for 20 nights were Dr. R. P. Cooke, a 26-year-old Acting Assistant Surgeon from the United States (Smith, 2019), and two American privates from the Hospital Corps, none of whom had previously been infected with yellow fever. It was reported that "All had remained in perfect health, notwithstanding their stay of twenty nights amid such unwholesome surroundings" (Reed, 1902).

In subsequent experiments in the same building, the researchers added greater exposure to fomites, including mattresses that yellow fever patients had slept on and by having the volunteers sleep in nightshirts that yellow fever patients had worn, and again found that the volunteers did not become sick. In the final round, the volunteers slept on "pillows covered with towels that had been thoroughly soiled with the blood drawn from both the general and capillary circulation, on the first day of the disease, in the case of a well-marked attack of yellow fever" (Reed, 1902). Reed ultimately deemed that attempts to infect people with yellow fever in the fomite house "an absolute failure" (Reed, 1902; Reed & Carroll, 1900), suggesting that fomites were not the culprit.

The other arm of the study may have been marginally less "yucky" but ultimately proved to be a lot riskier and more successful, in Reed's terms. This second set of volunteers, who were also not immune to yellow fever, stayed in tents in a different part of the camp. They were "subjected, with their full consent, to the bites of mosquitoes" that had fed on the blood of yellow fever patients. Out of the 12 participants who were exposed to mosquito bites, 10 became infected with yellow fever within the known period of incubation of the disease (Reed, 1902). Walter Reed also noted that two others also became infected in a similar way, and, for all of these people, "recovery happily followed" (Reed, 1902).

Through this experiment—and contrary to their prior beliefs—Walter Reed's team proved that yellow fever was transmitted by mosquitoes. Although the virus the mosquitoes were carrying was not identified until 1927 (Staples & Monath, 2008), this research was pivotal for public health efforts to essentially eradicate yellow fever from many countries. The knowledge that mosquitoes transmitted yellow fever even helped make it possible for the United States to build the Panama Canal. Prior attempts by the French to build a canal in Panama had failed in part because so many workers became sick with and died from yellow fever. Based on the findings from the yellow fever experiments, the Americans brought in public health officials who quarantined anyone who was sick, fumigated the houses where people who had become infected lived along with the homes of their neighbors, and eliminated standing pools of water and other places where mosquitoes could breed near the construction sites (Sutter, 2016).

To achieve these tremendous public health advancements, the sacrifices asked of research participants were substantial. Because there was no cure for yellow fever, Walter Reed's research participants faced a high chance of death. Walter Reed was said to have volunteered for deliberate infection but was prevented from doing so because his team believed that older individuals were more likely to die from the disease (Mehra, 2009). The members of the Yellow Fever Commission directly grappled with the ethics of conducting such risky research. Their informed consent process involved a formal contract that was printed in English and Spanish, and participants received $100 in gold (Lederer, 2008). Participants were also paid double the amount if they became ill, for a total of $200 (which was more than most of them made in a year). Whatever they earned would be given to their beneficiaries if they died.

The people who volunteered for the study were reportedly motivated by the thought that they were likely to be infected with yellow fever anyway since they had moved to Cuba. Altruism was also a factor; one Private John Kissinger initially refused payment saying that he wanted to participate "solely in the interest of humanity and the cause of science." Kissinger did benefit from his participation by later being promoted to the role of hospital steward, along with receiving a gold watch and $115 in cash (Smith, 2019). While the contract that prospective participants signed did mention that one's life could be endangered, it stated that this danger was only "to a certain extent," and this risk was contrasted with the supposed certainty of becoming infected with yellow fever in daily life in Cuba (Rothman, 1991). The research team also cited the high background risk of yellow fever in Cuba as a justification for deliberate infection in that setting, noting that the relative risk of deliberate infection was therefore lower in Cuba than in other places. Additionally, members of the investigative team served as research participants. In fact, one of them, Jesse Lazear, died after deliberately exposing himself to infected mosquitoes. To honor him, the research team named a part of the research site Camp Lazear.

Although it is sometimes reported that no deaths occurred (Pierce, 2003), this is only true if one focuses on the later phase of experimentation. In other early experiments involving direct inoculation with mosquitoes, there were three deaths that involved a 25-year-old contract nurse from the United States named Clara Maass, and two Spanish immigrants named Antonio Carro and Cumpersino Campa (Chaves-Carballo, 2013). Despite having been exposed to many yellow fever patients in the past, Maass had not been infected and was eager to acquire immunity. She was exposed to infected mosquitoes five times before finally becoming infected. On the sixth try, she was exposed to mosquitoes who had fed on Juan Alvarez, a 13-year-old boy whose case was particularly virulent. These so-called *Alvarez mosquitoes* transmitted a strain that appears to have been more lethal than others, as they were also used in the experiments with the two other volunteers who died. Although Maass was later honored with a bronze plaque in the Havana hospital where she died and with the issuance of stamps in her honor from the Cuban and US Postal Services (Chaves-Carballo, 2013), it is not clear where Carro and Campa received similar recognition for their sacrifices. Additionally, some members of the team who served as participants suffered significant longer-term harms. For example, one volunteer experienced chronic nerve damage and was considered mentally and physically weaker after the trial (Chaves-Carballo, 2013).

This practice of enrolling members of the research team into the study as participants, often referred to as "self-experimentation," was not uncommon at the time. For example, in 1892, two scientists swallowed cultures of cholera bacteria. One developed mild diarrhea while the other had severe cholera, thereby proving the cause of the disease (Benyajati, 1966). Some researchers did not enroll themselves, but did enroll family members. In 1900, a researcher named Patrick Manson tested whether mosquitoes transmitted malaria. It is thought that he enrolled his son in his early experiments and later cured him by administering quinine (Manson, 1900). Manson was keen to avoid the limitations of prior research that had been inconclusive. Previous challenge trials had been conducted in Italy, where malaria was endemic, making it difficult to prove that the experimental technique was responsible for malaria transmission. Manson therefore decided to infect an individual in central London, reasoning as follows:

> It occurred to me, therefore, that if I repeated [the Italian] experiments in a more dramatic and crucial manner, that if I fed laboratory-reared mosquitos on a malarial patient in a distant country and subsequently carried the mosquitos to the centre of London, and there set them to bite some healthy individual free from any suspicion of being malarial, and if this individual within a short period of being bitten developed malarial fever and showed in his blood the characteristic parasite, the conclusion that malaria is conveyed by the mosquito would be *evident to every understanding, and could not possibly be evaded.* (Manson, 1900; emphasis added)

As will be discussed in Chapter 5 in relation to emerging infectious diseases and the COVID-19 pandemic, Manson's insight still rings true today. The dramatic and (sometimes deceptive) simplicity of challenge studies may have attracted early researchers with limited scientific methods at their disposal. It also helps explain why challenge studies have captured the public's imagination more than a century—and several global infectious disease outbreaks—later.

For a similar purpose, but with a much less rigorous design, challenge studies were hastily deployed during the global influenza pandemic of 1918–1920. At that time, the cause of influenza was unknown, and it was widely thought to be a bacterial infection rather than a viral one. Some scientists attempted to isolate the cause of influenza infection by taking sputum samples from sick patients and injecting them into research participants, presumably with their consent, though it is unclear whether and how carefully consent was obtained. As with other early challenge studies, there was little attention to the fact that samples taken from sick patients could have contained more than one type of pathogen. In other words, these scientists were not certain what they were injecting into research participants, and whether they were exposing them to more than one pathogen. While these scientists were widely recognized for their contributions (Schultz & Morens, 2009), criticism for their particular ethical lapses is hard to find.

Yet looking beneath the service of other challenge studies conducted in the early twentieth century reveals hints of ethical unease even amid the highest scientific acclaim. One example of this was the intentional infection of neurosyphilis patients with malaria as a form of treatment (referred to as "malariotherapy"). This type of challenge research was different from other studies because it was done with a therapeutic intent to benefit the patients themselves. Although Julius Wagner-Jauregg was awarded the Nobel Prize in Medicine for his use of malariotherapy to treat syphilis that had spread to the brain in 1927, his experiments were both ethically and scientifically problematic.

For centuries, causing patients to have fevers had been considered a likely cure for syphilis, so the idea of infecting people with malaria to induce fevers that would cure syphilis was plausible to the scientific community. Malariotherapy had a fatality rate of between 1% and 9%, depending on whether patients were selected in advance for being at low risk, and could also cause other serious complications such as liver damage, hallucinations or delirium, nausea, and chronic headaches. Additionally, mistakes in administration of the therapy led to increased deaths in some cases. Wagner-Jauregg did not publish this information, but, in one case, patients were infected with a more virulent strain of malaria (*Plasmodium falciparum* instead of *P. vivax*), and several died as a result. Patients with neurosyphilis were also unlikely to have the capacity to give fully informed consent to this treatment, given the advanced state of their disease and its impact on cognitive capacity (Jamrozik & Selgelid, 2020). Strikingly, only one member of the Nobel Prize committee had reservations about awarding the prize to someone who had conducted such ethically troubling research. Wagner-Jauregg explained that the committee member indicated that "he would not be able to decide to award the Nobel Prize to a doctor who inoculated a paralytic with malaria, because he would be a criminal in his eyes." The prize was not awarded to Wagner-Jauregg until this committee member retired. In the end, it is remarkable that it remains unknown whether malariotherapy is effective because Wagner-Jauregg's research failed to control for confounding factors, making it hard to determine whether the treatment was curative, and we now have safer and more effective therapies for syphilis that render this question moot (Austin et al., 1992).

When (Some) Challenge Studies Began to Shock the World

The tide began to turn against challenge studies after egregiously unethical challenge studies were conducted during World War II. As noted above, despite the existence of regulations governing challenge studies, scientists working for the Axis powers used this research method in egregiously unethical ways. Among the horrific acts carried out by Nazis in concentration camps and Japanese researchers with prisoners of war were experiments deliberately exposing inmates to pathogens such as anthrax, malaria, chlamydia, cholera, tetanus, and dysentery. Experimental subjects were sometimes vivisected and killed after being infected to assess what damage was done to their internal organs (Tsuchiya, 2008; Weindling, 2008). One Japanese scientist wrote about his role in the experiments conducted on Chinese prisoners of war. He gave five men experimental vaccines against diseases like the plague, then intentionally exposed them to plague bacteria and finally dissected them while they were alive. Some people were used to test agents for biological warfare, including by being tied to stakes while anthrax bombs were dropped around them (Tsuchiya, 2008).

Because many of the victims of these experiments were killed, the full extent of the atrocities remains unknown. Although the experiments were ostensibly designed to develop scientific knowledge to benefit Nazi soldiers, the design of these studies suggests they were not driven entirely by scientific objectives but also to torture people who were considered less than human. The methods were typically not rigorous enough to produce meaningful data. Subjects in these experiments were exposed to incredibly high risks of death or serious disability without their voluntary consent.

The horrors of challenge studies conducted by German and Japanese scientists were revealed to the world when the physicians involved in these experiments were tried at the Nuremberg tribunal. The judges at the tribunal laid out 10 principles of medical research ethics that became the Nuremberg Code, a foundational document in research ethics.

While some of its principles have withstood the test of time better than others, the Nuremberg Code remains highly influential. The drafters of the Nuremberg Code began by stating that informed consent for research was essential for ethical research (Nuremberg Military Tribunals, 1949). Yet subsequent codes of ethics have diverged from Nuremberg and recognized research can be ethical even if it is conducted with people who cannot consent for themselves, such as children. Parental or surrogate permission could serve to protect their interests. Moreover, without research that addresses the needs of these groups, they are subject to ad hoc experimentation while receiving treatments or prophylaxis that had not been systematically tested and shown to be safe and effective for them.

Another part of the Nuremberg Code that was not adopted by other guidelines relates to limits on research risks. The Code indicated that risky research with an a priori chance of death or disabling injury should only be conducted if the researchers themselves participate.

This provision is widely believed to have been included to avoid condemning Walter Reed's yellow fever studies (Miller & Joffe, 2009), but it is not viewed as necessary or even ethically beneficial today. While some researchers on Reed's team did expose themselves to yellow fever, this is hardly the only way to distinguish their work from the egregiously unethical studies conducted during World War II.

Yet it is instructive that Nazi defendants in the Nuremberg trial sought to defend themselves by arguing that their horrific acts were similar to other experiments conducted around the same time. Researchers in the United States conducted challenge studies with influenza, dysentery, gonorrhea, and measles, among other pathogens, as part of the war effort. Perhaps the most famous example—and the one discussed at the Nuremberg trial—involved malaria challenge experiments. Some malaria challenge studies were conducted at Manteno State Hospital in Illinois with patients suffering from psychosis, who were unlikely to have the capacity to consent for, or even complain about, what was done to them. Others were conducted at Stateville Penitentiary, also in Illinois and known as Joliet Prison, between 1944 and 1946. In these trials, about 500 subjects were deliberately infected with malaria through mosquito bites or injections in order to test novel treatments. One incarcerated individual died from a heart attack as a result of participating in these studies. The Stateville experiments were featured in *Life* magazine, and a report from a state committee was even published in the *Journal of the American Medical Association* that declared these studies to be a model of ethical research. The studies enrolled incarcerated individuals who were asked for their informed consent, and not all of them elected to enroll in the research. Nevertheless, the carceral environment in which these studies were conducted was filled with different kinds of coercive measures. Additionally, some incarcerated people did not receive treatment for their symptoms until weeks after they started, raising questions about whether subjects were given the standard of care. The first dose of the experimental malaria drug given to prisoners was also the highest dose tolerated in monkeys, suggesting that risks were not minimized. While the Stateville Prison experiments were nowhere near as egregious as the Nazi experiments, they were still ethically problematic (Miller, 2013).

Ethically troubling challenge studies were also conducted by US investigators around the same time as the adoption of the Nuremberg Code in 1947. Researchers from the US government intentionally exposed vulnerable populations in Guatemala to sexually transmitted infections in the late 1940s without their understanding or consent. In these experiments, more than 1,300 incarcerated individuals, soldiers, and psychiatric patients were deliberately infected with syphilis, gonorrhea, and chancroid; fewer than half of them subsequently received treatment. Commercial sex workers were also sometimes intentionally infected and employed by the researchers to transmit disease to others. The researchers did not attempt to prevent transmission of infections to family members, despite the clear potential for transmission of syphilis to their wives or children. These studies only came to light decades after they were conducted. Soon after they were publicly revealed, President Obama tasked his Presidential Commission on Bioethics with reviewing these studies, and this commission referred to the research as "ethically impossible." Obama also formally apologized on behalf of the US government for its role in conducting these studies. The researchers conducting these experiments had conducted preliminary work to determine how to deliberately infect people with sexually transmitted infections in the federal penitentiary in Terre Haute, Indiana. In the United States, they set up procedures to obtain voluntary informed consent from participants. These researchers did not apply the same protections for participants in Guatemala, where they may have felt they could act with greater impunity (Presidential Commission, 2011).

Early Ethical Attention

In 1966, Henry Beecher published a canonical article in the *New England Journal of Medicine*, likely the earliest publication analyzing the ethics of challenge studies. Beecher detailed 22 examples of studies he deemed unethical, including an example of a challenge study conducted in institutionalized children (Beecher, 1966). He specifically called out research conducted at Willowbrook State School, a New York institution that housed approximately 6,000 intellectually disabled children (though it was originally designed to hold 3,000), in which these children were deliberately infected with hepatitis. Due to overcrowding and poor sanitation in the institution, hepatitis outbreaks occurred often. By 1954, nearly all children in the facility became infected within a year of arriving there (Faden & Beauchamp, 1986). A researcher named Saul Krugman was invited to the institution to study the outbreaks, with funding granted by the US Department of Defense. During his time at Willowbrook, Krugman performed several studies, including hepatitis challenge studies with children who lived there (Halpern, 2021).

Many ethicists have criticized the Willowbrook hepatitis studies, and they remain controversial. Beecher argued that the researchers had violated their duties as physicians to act in the interests of their patients and further that "[t]here is no right to risk an injury to one person for the benefit of others" (Beecher, 1966). Some ethicists have argued that these studies have faced unfair criticism, recognizing that Krugman was motivated to better understand and improve the conditions at Willowbrook. Given that most of the children in the institution were likely to become infected with hepatitis and that their symptoms were thought to be mild, the risk of being involved in these experiments was judged to be relatively low (Robinson & Unruh, 2008).

Some critics have raised the concern that parents of Willowbrook residents were coerced because they were waitlisted for placement at the institution—their children were offered a place at the research facility if the parents agreed to allow their children to participate in the research (Macklin & Sherwin, 1975). While parents seeking a place for their children at Willowbrook were not forced into having their children participate in the hepatitis challenge research (Robinson & Unruh, 2008), they may have had no reasonable alternatives. The research team gained an advantage from the challenging circumstances the parents were facing. In the 1950s and 1960s, institutional care was thought to be best for children with cognitive disabilities, and social support for families who cared for their children at home was very limited. It was also unclear that parents had enough information to understand the risks. Krugman himself admitted that the informed consent he obtained was "inadequate" at first, but said he made strides to improve the consent process by providing personal counseling to parents in 1964.

Krugman defended his research by comparing the risks of being infected in the study to the relatively high baseline risk of being infected in the institution and arguing that children benefitted by developing immunity (Krugman, 1986). Yet even if children had a relatively high chance of being infected through exposure to others at the institution, they were *certain* to be infected if enrolled in the research. Moreover, study participants were at increased risk of developing chronic liver disease down the road and did not necessarily receive protective doses of gamma-globulin to prevent their infection, unlike other residents at Willowbrook. Furthermore, the trials could have been conducted on the adult staff members working at Willowbrook, who were also at high risk of hepatitis. Krugman gave no compelling justification to conduct challenge studies with a doubly vulnerable population— children who were not able to give their own consent to research and who were also being raised in an institution apart from their families. Finally, since it was known at the time that unsanitary conditions led to higher rates of disease transmission, it is striking that the leadership at the institution chose to invest in bringing Krugman to the institution to conduct research on the causes of hepatitis rather than working to improve the sanitation and living conditions for the children who lived there. However, it may be that the problem was more structural than institutional and part of a much larger policy failure of underinvesting in the care of children with developmental disabilities.

Although Krugman's work has received a great deal of ethical attention, it was not conducted in isolation. In the book *Dangerous Medicine*, Sydney Halpern documents the oversight, direction, and support that Krugman received to conduct this research (Halpern, 2021). Furthermore, she chronicles three decades of hepatitis infection studies conducted with more than 3,700 individuals. One thousand of these individuals were exposed to hepatitis B and C, with an accompanying risk of becoming lifelong carriers. One hundred and fifty of the people exposed to hepatitis B in research studies were children. Krugman estimated that 800 children were involved in his studies, although most of these children were exposed to hepatitis A. Many of the adults in deliberate infection studies with hepatitis were incarcerated or housed in psychiatric institutions. Those who were exposed to hepatitis B or C, particularly as children, could have become lifelong carriers of the virus and passed it on to their children. At least 35 incarcerated individuals have been identified as having been exposed to hepatitis C. Both hepatitis B and C can lead to cirrhosis and liver cancer. Until relatively recently, treatments for hepatitis C were burdensome, had serious side effects, and were not curative for all patients, so these individuals may have had lifelong consequences from these experiments or even suffered early deaths as a result of their participation. Halpern notes that some researchers conducting these experiments attempted to advocate for their participants to receive life or disability insurance but were largely unsuccessful in securing resources for this purpose. The lack of a system to compensate injured research participants in the United States is a clear moral failing in this case and many others (Halpern, 2021). Coupled with a healthcare system that is inaccessible to many, this meant that many participants in these studies contributed to scientific advancement from which others would benefit, only to be left to carry the resulting harms and burdens by themselves.

Moving into the Modern Era

As public awareness of these controversies grew, fewer examples of challenge studies were published. Yet other examples of challenge studies were consistent with modern standards, even contemporaneously with some of the worst ethical violations. For instance, challenge studies with viruses causing the common cold, including certain coronaviruses, were conducted at the National Institutes of Health and the United Kingdom's Common Cold Unit beginning in the 1940s (Jamrozik & Selgelid, 2020). Additionally, an important shift in research regulation in the United States occurred in the 1970s, when the importance of research oversight became clear, and many past research abuses were brought to public attention.

Perhaps the most notorious research abuses in US history occurred in the Tuskegee syphilis study. Notably, this was not a challenge study. While the Tuskegee syphilis study did not involve deliberate human infection, to this day, many people believe that it did, including members of the press (Gale & Bloomberg, 2021). In fact, one qualitative study found that the myths about Tuskegee are, in some ways, more important than what transpired in the research. As one participant expressed, "And I think that over time the legend of Tuskegee is more palpable than what people know about what went down. I think I've always known. But I've always known that the government gave people syphilis, and this is not true" (Scharff et al., 2010).

Although they did not deliberately infect participants with syphilis, what researchers did in the Tuskegee Syphilis study was clearly unethical. This study was conducted by researchers within the US Public Health Service who followed Black men with syphilis for decades, without offering them treatments that were proven effective and became available over the course of the study. The legacy of the Tuskegee syphilis study still echoes today and may be a source of distrust toward medicine and research in the United States.

Despite these legitimate worries, the public outcry about Tuskegee and other unethical research has had profound consequences on the review and conduct of research today. The US Congress addressed public concern about research by creating a National Commission for the Protection of Subjects in Biomedical Research to lay the foundation for regulations governing research (U.S. Department of Health and Human Services, 1979). The federal regulations based on the work of the National Commission now require prior Institutional Review Board (IRB) review for research, assessment of risks and benefits, and obtaining written informed consent in most cases. While research oversight cannot prevent all research abuses (Kiernan, 1996; Sanmukhani & Tripathi, 2011), subsequent challenge studies tended to be much more controlled and did not enroll vulnerable populations. As will be discussed in subsequent chapters, there are now decades of experience for the safe use of many different types of CHI research in the modern era (Roestenberg et al., 2018).

Conclusion

Examining the history of challenge studies reveals their promise and peril simultaneously. Challenge studies have generated important scientific insights and public health achievements. Yet it is helpful to view these advances against the background of their long, complicated history. Recurring themes emerge through this examination of historical research.

First, although some results from CHI research have been scientific breakthroughs, CHI research is rarely transformative on its own. Revisiting the long experience with this controversial method reveals that CHI research has been used in prior pandemics long before the advent of modern safeguards for research. Yet some of the most significant results that challenge studies have produced in the past were related to fundamental scientific insights about disease transmission. As powerful as these findings can be, they must ultimately be incorporated into other trials and public policy to make an impact on the public's health. Challenge studies can be deceptively simple, and certain uses of challenge studies carry the potential for findings that are "evident to every understanding" (Manson, 1900). As we will see in Chapter 5, the ease of explaining some of the things that challenge studies can do may explain the outsize attraction of these studies to members of the public that was apparent in the widespread coverage of challenge studies during the COVID-19 pandemic.

It is also notable that the potential longer-term consequences of deliberate infection with pathogens often went unnoticed and unaddressed. Researchers conducting challenge studies did not always know what they were infecting participants with or how particular diseases can cause harm over time. In the absence of a legal requirement to compensate participants for research related injury, and with several barriers to recovering damages for injury in the tort system (Pike, 2012), people who contribute to science can be left to deal with long-term harms and burdens on their own. It is important that modern-day CHI research is conducted in ways that can ensure participants will have access to care if they are left with long-term injuries, such as compensation programs or by conducting CHI research in countries with universal healthcare.

Perhaps the clearest takeaway is the potential for abuse of this research method, particularly in the absence of robust oversight. Several studies were ethically troubling because they took unfair advantage of groups who were particularly vulnerable to exploitation, such as people who were incarcerated and children, and exposed them to shockingly high research risks. Selecting groups at a high baseline risk of infection was a common but problematic justification used by CHI researchers to involve people who were often ill-equipped to protect themselves or failed by the institutions that were supposed to care for them. In too many cases, investigators took advantage of existing injustices, neglected to attend to the underlying reasons that some people are at greater risk than others, and downplayed the risks to research subjects while inflating the societal benefits from their research. This has led to a protectionist ethic in research that has excluded many groups that have been categorized as vulnerable. In Chapter 6, we will return to this issue of how to address vulnerability to exploitation for CHI research participants without resorting to reflexive exclusion that can harm groups that are considered "vulnerable" by delaying or preventing their access to the benefits of research. Ultimately, understanding the many ways CHI research has been misused in the past will help lay a foundation for ethically sound uses of this research method in the future.

2

The "Yuck Factor"

Is Controlled Human Infection Research Intuitively Unethical?

Q: What was your first reaction to the idea of a COVID-19 infection study?
A: It seemed on its face to be unethical.
—Interview of a volunteer for 1 Day Sooner

Perhaps the most common first response to the idea of one person deliberately exposing another to a pathogen—and especially if it is a doctor deliberately infecting a patient—is that it is wrong to infect a healthy person (Vaz et al., 2021). This immediate reaction that controlled human infection (CHI) research is unethical seems to occur prior to rational assessment and not be based on specific concerns about the ethics of the research per se, which will be explored in Chapter 3. Such a reaction may lead some to rapidly conclude that CHI research is unethical, a response that seems to be grounded in instinct rather than reason.

One way to understand this reaction is through the so-called *yuck factor*, a term that sounds colloquial but that has been introduced and debated in the academic literature. Some ethicists, including Leon Kass and Art Caplan, have argued that the "yuck factor" reflects an intuitive reaction of disgust that can clue us into something that is morally wrong, while others disagree. There is a fundamental debate about whether the "yuck factor" is a source of moral insight. In this chapter, I delve into the debate on whether the "yuck factor" provoked by CHI research is worth taking seriously as a source of moral insight. I demonstrate that the "yuck factor" can be a useful signal for identifying ethical issues but is only of limited value in the ethical analysis of CHI research for two main reasons.

Intentionally Infecting Humans. Seema K. Shah, Oxford University Press. © Seema K. Shah 2026.
DOI: 10.1093/9780197667927.003.0002

First, empirical evidence suggests that the emotion of disgust is the product of evolutionary processes designed to avoid pathogens that could make us sick. If the root of disgust is an instinctual reaction to protect people from getting sick, there is no good reason it would align with considered moral judgment. Second, I show that different types of research invoke different levels of "yuck" responses but not in ways that mirror the level of moral concern that should accompany them, suggesting that this reaction may not be a useful signal for when moral concern is warranted. It would be a mistake to simply dismiss the "yuck factor," however. If there is a common, negative reaction to CHI research by members of the public that is related to the "yuck factor," it could lead to difficulty in recruiting for CHI research and generating support for it. Another explanation for this intuitive reaction is that it could be a form of shock or surprise that a medical professional is deliberately making someone sick in seeming violation of their moral duties. I discuss that issue in Chapter 3. In this chapter, I analyze the "yuck factor" in relation to CHI research and conclude that it is not a reliable source of moral wisdom. Nevertheless, the potential for such reactions to occur should spur greater attention to the community engagement that may be needed in advance of conducting types of CHI research that are likely to elicit a "yuck" reaction.

The "Yuck Factor"

In the late nineteenth century, Charles Darwin wrote about the emotion of disgust as a byproduct of evolution. He hypothesized that disgust had evolved to protect humans from rotten food that could cause disease (Darwin, 1872). The emotion of disgust came to take on moral salience in the ethics literature roughly 100 years later. Bioethicist Art Caplan is thought to have been the first to use the term "yuck factor" in 1994, as he described how the public might intuitively react to new scientific developments.

Leon Kass, a physician who later chaired George W. Bush's President's Council on Bioethics, expanded this idea and applied the concept to criticize human cloning (Schmidt, 2008). Kass famously argued that this instinctive reaction illustrates something morally important—what he called the "wisdom of repugnance" (Kass, 1998). Importantly, Kass acknowledged that people can be disgusted by a practice without good moral reasons, particularly if the reaction arises from prejudice or unfamiliarity. For example, so-called interracial marriage is something there is no good moral reason to oppose but that was once considered morally wrong by the dominant culture in the United States and in many countries around the world (and may still be for some people). Kass considered such examples as prejudice merely disguised as morality. However, he did not provide a principled way to separate things that mistakenly trigger our moral intuitions from truly immoral practices. He argued that the "yuck" reaction is important because it can alert us to deep moral truths, and that people can intuitively (or at least quickly) identify when their intuition is just misfiring.

Kass focused on human cloning as an example of when this "yuck" reaction gets it right. He argued that people react with revulsion to the prospect of human cloning "not because of the strangeness or novelty of the undertaking, but because we intuit and feel, immediately and without argument, the violation of things that we rightfully hold dear" (Kass, 1998). In other words, Kass saw the "yuck" reaction as a signal of a potential violation of the moral code to which one adheres. Kass's view that one just knows when something is unethical is hard to square with the fact that things that have widely been considered immoral in certain times and places are now commonly recognized to raise no moral concerns. Consider, for example, gay marriage. We now recognize that the "yuck" reaction many people likely felt toward homosexuality in the 1950s and 1960s in the United States was discriminatory, cruel, and morally wrong. Yet it is likely that many of those people felt it was a "violation of things"—such as the idea that marriage should only occur between a man and a woman—that they "rightfully held dear." Kass's view, then, fails to provide guidance about when a dominant view in a culture or society is morally wrong. Ideally, a moral account of CHI research would be able to provide guidance over time and across different contexts, which makes Kass's version of the "yuck factor" unhelpful for our purposes.

A more fundamental critique of this "yuck reaction" relates to its origins. For example, Martha Nussbaum is a prominent philosopher who has critiqued Kass's view because she identifies a different source for the "yuck reaction"—she sees it as stemming from the fear of one's own mortality (Nussbaum, 2004b). Nussbaum argues that the emotion of disgust typically focuses on reminders of our frailty and embodiment, and the "yuck" reaction that results is an attempt to manage this terror by recoiling so that we are prevented from having to think too deeply about it. Nussbaum is skeptical that this attempt to manage terror associated with mortality is useful for making moral or legal distinctions, arguing, "Does disgust, then, contain a wisdom that steers law in the right direction? Surely, the moral progress of a society can be measured by the degree to which it separates disgust from dangers and indignation, basing laws and social rules on substantive harm, rather than on the symbolic relationship an object bears to our anxieties" (Nussbaum, 2004a).

While Nussbaum's argument that it is unclear whether disgust points "in the right direction" is well taken, others have disagreed with her explanation for why we have a "yuck" reaction in the first place, bringing empirical evidence to bear on the question. In his book, *Yuck*, Daniel Kelly conducts an in-depth examination of empirical research on the "yuck factor" and then considers whether the emotional reaction of disgust tracks moral judgments (Kelly, 2011). Like Nussbaum, Kelly is skeptical that the "yuck factor" tracks morally relevant considerations. Kelly rejects Nussbaum's explanation for the origins of the "yuck reaction," however, explaining that it is inconsistent with empirical data about how disgust operates and the evolutionary pressures that must have led to its adoption. He notes that existing data support Darwin's early hypothesis that disgust initially evolved to keep us from eating rotten food that could make us sick. Yet Kelly explains how this emotion can be linked to moral and social norms. As I demonstrate, empirical explanations for the "yuck factor" are helpful for understanding why CHI research seems "yucky" *and* why some CHI research seems "yuckier" than others, so these explanations are worth examining it in greater detail.

Kelly argues that disgust is an emotion that operates on a "hair trigger" to keep humans (and other animals) away from poisons and parasites. This emotion errs on the side of false positives to maximize safety. He cites the ingestion of fecal matter as perhaps the paradigm example of something that elicits a strong response of disgust. This reaction is commonly associated with a "gape" face that resembles the start of gagging or vomiting; this facial expression has been shown to occur in both humans and primates. Over time, Kelly argues that this "yuck" reaction became co-opted to help regulate complex human interactions, including the creation and policing of social norms.

While Kelly contends that it is implausible that there is any way to nail down a single characteristic that we find disgusting, given the many different types of things that elicit disgust and the variability of the "yuck reaction" across people and cultures, he suggests there are common themes that can be sorted into categories of objects that elicit a reaction of disgust. First, disgust can be associated with signs of disease or phenotypic abnormalities in people—although this obviously can also be expressed in terms of prejudice against people who seem to be different. Second, disgust can be associated with food that people ingest, living animals that people associate with death (e.g., maggots, flies), and activities and fluids associated with sexual activity. There is, of course, variation in how different stimuli can elicit a "yuck" reaction—for example, which foods are disgusting varies a great deal by culture.

Kelly also argues that there is a common theme in disgust reactions to breaches of some social norms, particularly if the social norms involve something that is considered disgusting based on the evolutionary pathways mentioned above (like a corpse, for instance). There is one final class of norms that appears to have become unmoored from the evolutionary origins of the emotion—the violation of norms that relate to group membership. He gives the examples of Republicans and Democrats in the United States having disgust reactions toward each other or various policies or positions. Kelly asserts this reaction has been co-opted to enforce social—and moral—norms. One striking example of this is that one lab exposed participants to a wide variety of disgusting objects, including things that were classically disgusting and related to fecal matter. Researchers found that the object that provoked the most disgust was a sweater that had been worn by Adolf Hitler.

Kelly marshals considerable empirical data to support these claims, such as studies using functional magnetic resonance imaging (MRI) technology that demonstrate that the same patterns of neural activity occur when people are provided with descriptions of others doing things like "eating a scab" and also when they are informed about sociomoral violations like incest (Schaich Borg et al., 2008). Kelly concludes that disgust should be understood as a byproduct of a system that worked when protecting people from contamination, but one that may not work well when pressed into service to make moral judgments (Kelly, 2011). For example, Kelly provides evidence that there is a strong contamination effect from anything associated with something considered disgusting, and it is easier to contaminate something than to render it safe again. To wit: one drop of feces is sufficient to contaminate one bottle of wine, and even adding enough wine to fill a cask would still elicit disgust and unwillingness to consume it.

Other studies attempting to understand the evolutionary origins of disgust, and specifically disgust as a sensitivity to pathogens, have noted that there are contextual reasons that disgust manifests more in some contexts than others. The emotion of disgust is a bit of a luxury. In lower-income societies, where dirt floors are the norm, a strong disgust reaction to dirt and related pathogens would make it difficult to function. Thus, the emotion is most useful if one has the means to avoid pathogens in the first place. Additionally, the emotion of disgust in response to pathogens might be more adaptive in countries or settings with more pathogens. There is reason to think that the emotion of disgust adapts to context and is able to protect people against disease in some contexts, thus providing an evolutionary advantage.

With such evidence supporting his theory of disgust, Kelly argues forcefully against Nussbaum's theory that disgust is connected to the terror we feel when faced with our own mortality. Like Nussbaum, however, Kelly is skeptical of the connection between disgust and moral wisdom. For his part, Kelly demonstrates this with examples of extreme prejudice, such as how Nazis conceived of Jewish people prior to and during World War II and biases within the caste system in India (Kelly, 2011). For example, traditional Brahmins in India hold the belief that if a person of lower caste uses their kitchen to cook food, the kitchen will become contaminated and cannot be used until it is cleansed. This belief is rooted in prejudice and oppression and not based on some natural moral wisdom. As Kelly puts it, "one of the most prominent functions that disgust has come to play in our [Western] putative moral psychology is to support decidedly *immoral* attitudes" (Kelly, 2011). This may be one of the most important points Kelly makes, and one that has surprising relevance to CHI research, as we will see below.

Indeed, there are prominent instances of people who overcame the normal reaction of disgust to perform morally praiseworthy acts by demonstrating care for people who had been unfairly stigmatized. For example, the late Princess Diana's decision to shake hands with people living with HIV/AIDS in the late 1980s, even though many believed erroneously at that time that HIV/AIDS could be spread through any form of direct physical contact, was widely lauded. Similarly, Fred Rogers took a stand against views that it was wrong for Black people and White people to share public pools because of the racist belief that Black people were likely to spread disease. In 1969, Mr. Rogers invited Officer Clemmons, a black man who played a police officer on the beloved children's program called *Sesame Street*, to join him in cooling off his feet in a small inflatable pool, and both men shared a towel to dry off their feet afterward (Kettler, 2020). At that time, many public pools were segregated, and some cities resisted orders to integrate public pools by failing to maintain them so they could shut them down as a result of disrepair (Smith, 2012). Rogers took a moral stance against these immoral beliefs, unconcerned about whether racist viewers would find it triggered their personal, misfiring "yuck factors."

Notably, Kelly's theory does not resolve all of the puzzles that the emotion of disgust and the "yuck" reaction raises. While agreeing that disgust is "an emotion whose principal function is to help us avoid contaminants and disease—a kind of behavioral extension of the immune system," Nina Strohminger points out many unanswered questions about disgust that suggest it is highly complex. In an excoriating and entertaining book review, Strohminger points out the limitations of some theorists of disgust, including that they ignore the enjoyment or allure of disgust, such as that experienced by viewers of a "gory zombie movie" (Strohminger, 2014b). Strohminger also points out that "the veneration of sexual purity" is related to disgust but "touches on moral, mating, and pathogenic concerns" that go beyond protection from disease (2014). She concludes that disgust is a multifaceted emotion that encompasses several different concepts, but, importantly for our purposes, one that may overlap with moral judgments (Strohminger, 2014b).

Ultimately, whatever one thinks of the evolutionary origins of disgust or the boundaries of this emotion, empirical evidence about the triggers of disgust can explain why CHI research elicits a "yuck" reaction. It also provides clues as to what makes some types of CHI research "yuckier" than other types, as will be discussed further below. When we apply this "yuck factor" to research, however, I demonstrate that it does not correlate with the features of research that make it morally problematic and sometimes attaches to CHI research that can be conducted ethically.

"Yucky" Controlled Human Infection Research

Strikingly, some features of CHI research are things that commonly elicit disgust. Perhaps most notably, all CHI research intentionally exposes individuals to pathogens, typically to cause infection. Certain examples of CHI research also seem almost like they were designed to elicit a strong reaction of disgust.

As discussed in the Introduction, CHI research is typically conducted with pathogens that cause three main categories of diseases: (1) enteric pathogens that infect the gut and digestive system and cause vomiting and diarrhea (such as cholera), (2) respiratory pathogens that attack the lungs and circulatory system (think influenza or COVID-19), and (3) vector-borne diseases that are typically transmitted by mosquitoes, ticks, and other vectors (which, in cases like Zika virus, can include sexual transmission and transmission from a pregnant person to a fetus or newborn). For respiratory viruses, which have now become much better understood by the public due to the COVID-19 pandemic, particles can be aerosolized so participants can inhale the pathogen, or droplets containing viruses can be placed with a pipette into the nostril directly. Aerosolizing particles is closer to how people are infected in the real world, but in cases where researchers are worried about having members of their team infected, as with CHI models to address COVID-19, placing virus particles into the nostril directly is the favored approach. CHI research involving enteric pathogens, such as CHI studies with *Salmonella typhoid*, commonly requires participants to drink a sludge containing the bacteria that infects them (McNeil Jr, 2017). The particles can come from various fluids that include infectious particles obtained from sick people, including fecal matter. Yet not everyone finds the idea of drinking a fluid that contains high levels of a pathogen found in fecal matter disgusting. One volunteer described their experience participating in a CHI that required drinking a solution containing typhoid as follows: "It was all quite underwhelming. It was served in a typical laboratory tube. I expected it to taste more 'typhoidy.' Not like poop, that is—the things that make poop smell like poop are absolutely different bacterially. But I expected something. A lot of cultures have a typical smell. It was clear, I think, and it tasted like nothing particular."[1]

There is also some CHI research that does not fall into any of these categories. For example, CHI research with hookworm requires exposure to parasitic worms. In CHI research with schistosomiasis, researchers create a liquid full of worms that they place on a patch that goes onto participants' wrists. The worms burrow through a person's skin, travel through the bloodstream to the lungs, and ultimately attach themselves to the lining of the small intestine, where they can survive as parasites (Murphy, 2018). Recall also that exposing people to pathogens can also happen in different ways. For example, some controlled human malaria infection studies involve using a syringe filled with malaria parasites to inject participants intravenously with the disease-causing agent, whereas others involve placing a cup of infected mosquitoes on the arms of participants until they have been bitten (Stanisic et al., 2018).

Finally, there are also examples of "challenge trials" related to mental health that do not expose participants to pathogens but instead attempt to provoke psychiatric symptoms. Consider, for example, trials exposing participants to carbon dioxide or a stimulus about which they have a phobia to trigger a response like panic attacks or obsessive-compulsive symptoms. Frank Miller and Don Rosenstein have examined what they call "psychiatric symptom-provoking"

---

[1] https://www.nytimes.com/2017/09/28/health/typhoid-vaccine-trial.html.

studies (Miller & Rosenstein, 1997). These studies typically also involve measuring physiological and biochemical changes in the body in response to the challenge. These studies can be used for several purposes, including to help understand the pathophysiology behind the disorders, distinguish between similar but distinct conditions, and help develop new diagnostic tests and treatments. For example, psychiatric symptom-provoking studies have been used to establish that panic disorder and obsessive-compulsive disorder are different from each other.

While most symptoms experienced by participants in these studies are transient and similar to what the patients commonly experience, they can raise serious risks. For example, one study tested whether causing people to have panic attacks made them more likely to have panic attacks in response to the same stimuli in the future (Yeragani et al., 1988). In another study of Vietnam veterans who were given infusions of lactate to provoke symptoms of post-traumatic stress disorder, all of the participants became depressed and felt guilty during flashbacks, and one experienced severe distress: "Patient 7 burst into tears during a lactate flashback as he saw his best friend blown up by a booby-trapped grenade" (Rainey et al., 1987). These studies clearly can raise ethical concerns that we will return to in Chapter 3, but, for present purposes, they may not raise the same type of a visceral "yuck" reaction as a study that involves drinking a sludge made from fecal matter that contains parasitic worms.

Indeed, some of these examples evoke a greater "yuck" reaction than others, or even two different kinds of "yuck" reactions, such as the challenge trials with malaria conducted by Nazis mentioned in Chapter 1. Yet there is an inherent subjectivity to "yuckiness"; some things that may seem "yucky" to some people are less so to others. For instance, one might think that the idea of having someone placing a cup of malaria-infected mosquitoes on one's arm would elicit disgust from potential participants. When we conducted a qualitative study with participants in controlled human malaria infection studies, however, most participants were not bothered by having the cup of mosquitoes placed on their arm, with only one exception. Some people said that they had spent their summers getting bitten by mosquitoes while on Lake Michigan, so they were unperturbed by the experience.

The only person who expressed some irritation about it was a participant who had to sit through five different cups of mosquitoes before they found one that would bite him (Kraft et al., 2019). Admittedly, the 16 participants who agreed to enroll in this small study were likely self-selected for those who were less bothered by mosquito bites. It is telling, however, that there are people for whom the process of being infected by malaria by allowing themselves to be feasted on by mosquitoes does not seem disgusting.

By contrast, consider the examples of drinking sludge prepared with fecal matter from sick people or having a patch of parasitic worms placed onto your skin to cause infection. The disgust one experiences in contemplating these examples could be focused on either the act of physical contact with something that is disgusting or the fact that people are being infected with diseases on purpose, or both. And the disgust that is connected to the former—contact with something disgusting—is not a moral form of disgust at all. It is, rather, about how gross that thing is. This, too, varies across people: consider the quote of the participant in a typhoid CHI model who did not find it disgusting to ingest a solution derived from fecal matter.

Kelly's analysis also suggests that there is also a third and more subtle type of disgust that could be linked to challenge studies—one that is socially mediated. Historical challenge studies sometimes involved serious moral violations. In particular, many of the examples discussed in Chapter 1, and the challenge studies conducted by the Nazis in particular, are examples that many members of the public may still associate with challenge studies being conducted today. Thus, while some of the disgust reaction elicited by CHI research can be explained by the evolved reaction to avoid contamination and disease, it is also possible that challenge studies in general have been contaminated by their association with unethical research conducted in the past.

Furthermore, historical violations may be stickier than other associations and possibly easier for people to bring to mind. As noted above, the "yuck" reaction easily contaminates objects. People are also better at remembering things if they are disgusting (Charash & McKay, 2002; Kelly, 2011). People are likely to hold on to their belief that something is wrong or disgusting even when they can give no defensible reasons for why they believe this. This suggests that urban legends that invoke the disgusting elements of CHI research may be more likely to spread.

One prominent example of this may be the widespread misconception that the subjects of the Tuskegee syphilis studies were deliberately injected with syphilis, rather than realizing these men were unethically denied access to or knowledge about treatment for syphilis after being infected naturally. Recall the example from Chapter 1 of the individual who said he knew that the men in the Tuskegee syphilis study were deliberately infected with syphilis, even though he also knew that they weren't. For a member of the public who does not spend a lot of time thinking about research in general or CHI research in particular, some of these judgments may be relatively impervious to reasons, particularly if they remain unexamined or uncontested.

It seems clear that the "yuck" factor is unlikely to be a source of clear moral wisdom in a rigorous ethical analysis of CHI research. It is possible, however, that the "yuck" factor is a signal that alerts us to the possible presence of ethical issues in a way that is worth investigating further. In Chapter 3, we will explore whether there is anything ethically unique about CHI research and use that to develop an ethical framework for CHI research in Chapter 4. Before addressing the unique ethical issues that may or may not arise in CHI research, however, it is important to examine whether CHI research uniquely generates a "yuck" response or if other research might do so as well.

"Yucky" Research in General

While challenge studies might elicit a "yuck reaction" in many people, they are far from the only type of research that triggers the "yuck reaction." For example, consider research (1) involving brain dead individuals, (2) in which participants are studied while having sexual intercourse, or (3) involving the amputation and reattachment of toes. By examining these types of studies, it becomes clear that the "yuck factor" does not help us in evaluating whether research is ethically appropriate.

For example, one study involved the transplantation of kidneys from genetically modified pigs to two people who were determined to be brain dead. After transplantation, the recipients of the organ were kept on respirators for 54 hours to see if the kidneys worked. The experiment was successful. There was no evidence of the human bodies rejecting the pig kidneys, and the pig kidneys functioned better than the original kidneys, even producing urine (Montgomery et al., 2022). At the end of the article, the authors indicate the next step is to test whether a genetically modified pig kidney could last in a brain dead person's body for longer periods of time. While there is legitimate controversy over whether brain death is a form of biological death or a social or legal construction—even setting that controversy aside—this type of research might evoke a "yuck" reaction from many people who feel it is intuitively wrong to desecrate corpses (DeVita et al., 2003).

But is this yuck reaction telling us anything of moral importance? Many ethicists would say no. Ethicists have argued that research with people determined to be dead under neurological criteria can be done ethically (DeVita et al., 2003). If someone has given their voluntary informed consent to donate their body to science, why is it more ethically acceptable to wait until their heart has stopped beating to enroll them in such research? Particularly if that person expressed an interest in certain types of research, it could be ethically beneficial to their legacy or the sense that they contributed to something important (Wendler, 2010). One concern might be that the interests of brain dead patients are more easily overlooked. To address the (unlikely) possibility that brain dead people might still feel pain, participants could still be anesthetized before the surgery was performed. Another question might arise about whether the research has enough social value to justify conducting it. The value of this research seems compelling because of critical organ shortages around the world. If organs could be cultivated in animals, tens of thousands of lives could be saved each year in the United States alone. While some might initially balk at the thought of receiving a pig liver, few people would turn it down if it was a choice between life and death, and some patients have willingly taken the gamble of receiving these organs (Montgomery et al., 2022).

A similar example of potentially "yucky" research is the Last Gift study, which was designed to study a critical, unanswered question that makes it difficult to find a cure for HIV (Riggs et al., 2022). In this study, people living with HIV who are nearing the ends of their lives agree to have their bodies undergo rapid autopsies as soon as possible after they are pronounced dead. The goal of the autopsies is to find the reservoirs where HIV hides in the body that antiretroviral drugs cannot reach. If these viral reservoirs can be identified, this will make it easier to one day develop an approach to eradicating HIV from an individual's body to cure them of the disease. The Last Gift study raised many ethical issues, but it is not clear that the "yuck" reaction should suggest that this study was uniquely problematic. Furthermore, diagnosing ethical issues is different from determining whether they can be addressed. The team conducting this study included an ethicist who helped guide the responses to both anticipated and unanticipated issues (Kanazawa et al., 2023). None of the issues identified seemed to be unique to this study, however. For example, one anticipated concern was that patients would conflate involvement in the research with provision of clinical care and misunderstand the purpose of the research. This was addressed by ensuring that the study did not offer clinical care, and any study staff who might have been involved in a patient's care were not allowed to perform research procedures on that patient. Another issue arose when a participant was friends with one of the study nurses prior to enrolling in the study. The participant and the nurse were asked about whether they would prefer to interact in the study or not, and they both found comfort in working with each other. This agreement was periodically revisited to ensure that appropriate boundaries were in place, and both the nurse and the participant continued to feel comfortable with the arrangement.

Another famous example of research that might induce a "yuck" response was conducted by William Masters and Virginia Johnson, who conducted several direct observation studies of people having sexual intercourse in their laboratory. While Masters and Johnson undoubtedly crossed ethical and legal lines, particularly related to consent, some of their studies were arguably not ethically problematic. For instance, they did conduct several studies of married couples having sexual intercourse in the lab while connected to a series of wires and instruments to measure different physiologic responses. Through these studies, they were able to generate groundbreaking insights about sexual activity (Greenberg et al., 2013). The idea of scientists paying married couples to have sexual intercourse while being observed and connected to wires and instruments may seem "yucky" to many and is likely not what most people think of when they imagine biomedical research. Nevertheless, if participants gave their consent, and the risks were minimized and determined to be acceptable, these studies are not necessarily wrong or unethical.

There are also activities outside of the research context that raise the "yuck factor," such as "chickenpox parties" and reality television shows that require participants to engage in behaviors that elicit disgust. Following the COVID-19 pandemic, some parents who are worried about vaccination and more comfortable with exposures they see as natural have held "chickenpox parties." This practice is common enough that the Centers for Disease Control and Prevention has issued a warning against having such parties, explaining that the consequences can be very serious and that vaccination is a safer alternative for inducing immunity in children (Centers for Disease Control and Prevention, 2024). One interesting feature of this example is that some parents do not find it objectionable. Infectious disease physician and ethicist Zeb Jamrozik has even argued that such parties are actually preferable to nonvaccination (even if vaccination would be the best option) and provides criteria for an ethical chickenpox party: (1) the disease is low risk for most children, (2) parents give their consent, and (3) children who are infected quarantine for enough time to prevent spreading the disease to others (Jamrozik, 2018).

Chickenpox parties are a good example, then, of a situation that is not universally "yucky" and could arguably be ethically justified under certain circumstances. For example, when vaccinations against smallpox were not available in the 1800s, inoculation with the virus was a common and ethically defensible practice in young children to reduce mortality and the disfigurement associated with the disease. It seems that deliberate exposure through "chickenpox parties" is not morally objectionable on its face but rather in comparison to the safer alternative of vaccinating one's children. Thus, deliberate exposure outside of the research context is considered acceptable by many and is not ethically objectionable per se, even if it could be problematic in particular cases.[2] Yuckiness, then, does not tell us much about how to diagnose when something is ethically problematic and when it is not.

Thus, other types of research and even some non-research activities also raise the "yuck" reaction, and CHI research is not unique in this respect. Across this wide variety of cases, however, it is not clear that the "yuck" reaction helps us in diagnosing or addressing ethical concerns. Anticipating that members of the public might have a "yuck" reaction could be important for one final reason, however—it may help to identify potential threats to public trust. The presence of "yuck" reactions may support Hope and McMillan's arguments that challenge studies may threaten the need to preserve public trust in research, and extra attention to this potential public reaction may be warranted.

Do Members of the Public Actually Find Controlled Human Infection Research "Yucky"?

Studies of public views on CHI research have only recently begun to emerge to shed light on whether some or all CHI research elicits the "yuck reaction." A handful of studies have been conducted to better understand the views of the public about CHI research, largely finding that CHI research is acceptable to participants, in theory, as long as ethical safeguards are in place (Barker et al., 2022; Egesa et al., 2022; Gordon et al., 2023; Mtunthama Toto et al., 2021; Piggin et al., 2022). One such study was conducted in advance of the UK's CHI research to address COVID-19 (Barker et al., 2022). In this study, 57 participants who were predominantly female and between the ages of 20 and 40 were involved in focus groups and asked about their perceptions of and concerns about a study deliberately infecting people with SARS-CoV-2. The researchers conveyed to participants that CHI research could help accelerate development of the initial COVID vaccines

---

[2] While beyond the scope of this book, it is interesting to consider whether the practice of exposing oneself to a disease after vaccination could be ethical. For example, many parents report allowing themselves to be exposed to COVID-19 if their children test positive, after having been vaccinated and boosted. This desire for control in the timing of illness is understandable even if it would not necessarily be recommended. This scenario is not entirely dissimilar from a "chickenpox party."

(even though this is not how CHI models with SARS-CoV-2 were ultimately used). The authors of this study noted that no one felt that the study should not be done—an interesting use of a double negative. While participants wanted the ultimate decision to be made by an ethics board, they noted that there should be "emphasis on this being a ground-breaking piece of research and all the people you could help, loads of emphasis on that," in making the judgment about whether the study should be done (Barker et al., 2022). This suggests that participants did not fully understand the complex ways that SARS-CoV-2 CHI research could contribute to social value. Keeping these limitations in mind, this study did not support a "yuck" reaction to the prospect of conducting CHI research among members of the public. Their concerns about risk were characterized as "significant personal anxiety" about the risk of severe disease or death, a fear mitigated for some people by the thought of getting infected in a controlled setting as opposed to being infected in an uncontrolled way in the real world.

To engage with a broader group, these authors next conducted online surveys with more than 2,400 people about the acceptability of CHI research with SARS-CoV-2 (Barker et al., 2022). Most participants (78%) did not know what a CHI study was before taking part in the survey. Many of the concerns raised were about risks and burdens, including long COVID and the potential impact on mental health of being in isolation for lengthy periods of time. The authors of this study pointed out that, although there was agreement among the survey participants that the study was worth doing, only 33% of respondents reported being willing to take part in such research themselves. Furthermore, several expressed concern about the idea of having their family members enrolled in SARS-CoV-2 CHI research. For instance, one person said, "My son falls into the age category where . . . he could be used as a volunteer, and I'd be absolutely terrified . . . it's that fear of someone who you're very close to potentially putting their life at risk." Notably, other qualitative studies about CHI research participation have found this same issue with a parent raising concerns about CHI research. For example, in a qualitative study of participants in a CHI study involving malaria, one participant said his mother offered to pay him the same amount of money he would make for enrolling in the CHI study if he did not participate. In that case, however, he chose to participate regardless (Kraft, 2018).

Another study seeking to understand public views on CHI models was conducted by researchers developing a CHI model for leishmaniasis (Parkash et al., 2021). Leishmaniasis is a disfiguring disease with a substantial disease burden that primarily affects people in lower-income countries. Cutaneous leishmaniasis causes sores around the body that can be difficult to treat. The disease is transmitted by sand fly bites, and research in mouse models suggested that vaccines that work against leishmaniasis that is injected into mice did not work as well against leishmaniasis that was transmitted by sand fly bites, thus suggesting that a CHI model in which people were infected with leishmaniasis by sand fly bites would have considerable value. Given the potential "yuck" reaction of the public to a CHI model involving exposing people to the bites of sand flies and a subsequent skin disease that could leave them with permanent scars, the researchers planning to develop this model decided to focus on engaging the public in advance of developing the model. They therefore enrolled 10 people in a qualitative study to better understand their views. Participants were largely supportive of the study once they understood why it was being conducted. They had some valuable and surprising suggestions for improvement. Some of these suggestions related to the informed consent process and how researchers should anticipate that participants might google the term "sand fly bite" and become deterred from participating, especially if they failed to realize that there were different types of sand flies and the bites they would receive in research would be relatively small. Participants also thought the purpose and potential value of the research was not sufficiently clear in the informed consent document.

One question that participants focused on was where the bite should occur. While the participants agreed that researchers should propose having the bite occur in the pit of the elbow, they felt it would be helpful to let participants choose a different location if they preferred another site. Additionally, researchers had ruled out the possibility of surgical removal of the lesion at the site of the sand fly bite as too risky, even though biopsy of the site would be valuable for research purposes to confirm infection. Participants, however, thought this was the best way to treat the bite, in comparison to options such as injecting medication into the site, especially because it added value to the research.

Another study was conducted by Vaz and colleagues to understand the potential acceptability of CHI research in India. No CHI research had been conducted in India at the time of the study (Vaz et al., 2021). Vaz and colleagues aimed to study "a cross-section of society" across age, gender, different types of occupations, and different religious and caste groups (although some participants from urban settings did not disclose their religion or caste). They conducted 11 focus groups, 5 in rural settings and 6 in urban settings, with between 6 and 11 participants in each one, for a total of 92 participants. (While not as important for present purposes, they also interviewed key informants who had relevant expertise.)

Focus group participants had difficulty understanding the potential benefits from CHI research. Of interest, one participant thought that an epidemic might be the only justification, arguing that "to save those many lives this action should be taken . . . until then I think this is not required." Participants asked whether CHI research was necessary given other ways to gather data, including by studying natural infection, but they did not rule out the conduct of CHI research in India. Some participants raised concerns about risks and compensation for long-term injury. For instance, one person was worried that "We also don't know the long-term repercussions, we actually don't know if the small virus is going to mutate, we want to know what the outcome is." Furthermore, there were concerns that the health system might fail to provide needed care for and be "non-responsive" to long-term effects. Participants also wanted to ensure voluntary informed consent and that high compensation did not make it likely that vulnerable groups would be exploited. Of note, the authors struggled with an important challenge to effective public engagement about CHI research. When conducting focus groups in India, they had difficulty in translating words like "ethics" and "controlled" into other languages, which made it harder for the lay public to understand these terms.

Conclusion

If certain types of CHI research are particularly likely to trigger the "yuck factor," what are the implications of this for research teams, research oversight groups, and policymakers? First, policymakers and members of research oversight committees should consider the potential "yuck factor" for a given study and ensure that when this potential is heightened, the study team is planning to address this issue directly. For instance, when CHI research with malaria was first planned to be conducted in Kenya, Dorcas Kamuya led a plan to address the fact that the conduct of CHI research "can give rise to increased rumors and jeopardize research participation in study activities" (Mumba et al., 2022). Kamuya and colleagues have undertaken in-depth community engagement work to dispel some of these concerns. As discussed at greater length in Chapter 6, this work includes the creation of an elected body of approximately 200 people who represent residents living in the area, with each person serving a 3-year term. Engagement sessions with this body revealed several concerns, including questioning why so much blood was taken for the study— some people even raised concerns that it might be linked to worship of the devil. The comprehensive engagement strategy also included embedded social science work to enable continued learning and adapting to changes. This example illustrates one way that researchers can thoughtfully plan in advance for conducting CHI research that is likely to elicit a "yuck reaction" to anticipate and address this reaction without giving unwarranted ethical credence to it. While such community engagement is critically important for practical reasons, there may also be moral reasons to do it that we have not yet examined. To fully address the ethical issues raised by CHI research requires first understanding what they are, and whether there is anything ethically unique about CHI research, as we turn to in the next chapter.

3

Is CHI Research Ethically Unique?

> *Q: What was your first reaction to the idea of a COVID-19 infection study?*
> *A: I think it's a brilliant idea. It's one of those rare times where I think the typical ethics rules should be inverted.*
> —Prospective volunteer who signed up for SARS-CoV-2 CHI research with 1Day Sooner

In this chapter, I examine whether there is anything ethically unique about controlled human infection (CHI) research. CHI research has been described as "ethically sensitive" (Jamrozik & Selgelid, 2020) or uniquely "morally problematic." But is CHI research morally unique, or is it no different from other types of research? Given the heated debate over CHI models in research to address COVID-19 (Eyal et al., 2020; Kahn et al., 2020; Shah et al., 2020), along with substantial interest in using CHI research in future pandemics and for other indications (Barnes et al., 2023), the question of whether CHI research is morally distinct deserves more attention than it has received. In this chapter, I attempt to isolate whether there are objective moral reasons to treat CHI research differently from other types of research or other activities, or whether misperceptions about CHI research along with misfiring intuitions—perhaps related to the "yuck factor" discussed in Chapter 2—simply makes it *feel* ethically distinct.

I begin by reviewing prior ethical debates about CHI research. Although some ethicists have argued that CHI research is not ethically unique, they have not focused enough on a crucial distinction within this type of research—the difference between models and studies. I will explain how CHI models are different when researchers truly venture into uncharted territory and set the parameters for what subsequent studies will do. This means that, as a general rule, CHI models

Intentionally Infecting Humans. Seema K. Shah, Oxford University Press. © Seema K. Shah 2026. DOI: 10.1093/9780197667927.003.0003

are more ethically distinct from other types of research and therefore require extra ethical attention.

I then investigate several potential ways that CHI research—particularly CHI models—might be unique from an ethical perspective. I demonstrate that CHI research is neither more risky nor more lucrative than other types of research. In other respects, however, CHI research is unusual. Although many of the unusual features of CHI research are not entirely unique and can be found in other such endeavors, CHI research is unusual because it presents a cluster of complex and/or unresolved issues.

Ultimately, I demonstrate that CHI research *sometimes* requires greater ethical attention because it can present a collection of five complex and/or unresolved ethical issues: (1) highly uncertain social value, (2) intentional infection of participants, (3) uncertain and potentially high risk for participants, (4) third-party risk, and (5) risks associated with early withdrawal from the study. These issues are compounded when CHI research with a high degree of uncertainty is being conducted, such as the creation of a new CHI model that has particularly uncertain social value and risk on its own and sets the parameters for future CHI studies by resolving these ethical issues in particular ways—for example, by selecting whether a widely-circulating or weakened strain of the pathogen will be used and determining whether and if so, for how long, participants will be confined. The fact that CHI research is ethically complex does not mean that it is always ethically questionable. Rather, this analysis will lay the groundwork for an ethical framework presented in Chapter 4 that lays out the processes to use and issues to address for CHI research to be ethically acceptable—which will also make clearer when CHI research crosses ethical red lines.

Is CHI Research Ethically Distinct from Other Types of Research?

Some ethicists who examined CHI research have noted that while it intuitively seems unique, it bears many similarities to other types of research. As noted previously, the first sustained treatment of the ethics of CHI research was published in 2001, by Frank Miller and Christine Grady. Miller and Grady focused on the net risks posed by CHI research to healthy volunteers and argued that "[i]nfection-inducing challenge experiments are not necessarily any more ethically problematic than are phase I trials aimed at the determination of the maximum tolerated doses of investigational agents. Such trials typically enroll healthy volunteers who are exposed to potential side effects and complications without any compensating medical benefits" (2001). A few years later, Hope and McMillan similarly concluded that CHI research is not ethically unique. Hope and McMillan acknowledged one important caveat: even if there is no morally relevant difference between CHI and other types of research, the public might react differently to CHI research than other types of research. Therefore, to preserve public trust in research, Hope and McMillan suggest there is a need for greater caution in conducting CHI research (2004). Importantly, this suggestion stemmed from worries about the public perception of CHI research, which, as discussed in the preceding chapter, may be supported by evidence about the "yuck reaction." The authors did not argue that members of the public were correct to believe that CHI research is morally unique, but that negative reactions are foreseeable and should be taken into account to ensure conducting CHI research does not threaten public trust—in other words, they saw it as a public relations issue more than an ethical concern.

In 2015, Bambery, Selgelid, Weijer, Savelescu, and Pollard took a slightly different approach (Bambery et al., 2015). While these authors agreed with Hope and McMillan's concern about public trust as a factor that distinguishes CHI research from other types of research, they also added additional considerations for why CHI research is ethically distinct from other research. Bambery and colleagues found it morally problematic that CHI researchers intend to infect participants *and* that there is a direct link between the researcher's actions and harm to participants. They also raised concerns about third-party risks that can occur if research participants spread diseases to others not enrolled in the study and argued that these risks deserve careful attention.

This concern about researchers' intentions has been shared by others. Anuradha Rose contends that "[i]n challenge studies potential harm experienced by participants is intended, not merely potentially foreseen, as in clinical trials that evaluate safety" (2018). And in a workshop involving experts from various disciplines about the acceptability of doing CHI research in India, participants concluded that "[t] he 'intention to harm by purposefully causing infection in a person makes a CHI model study different from a Phase 1 Clinical Trial which also recruits healthy volunteers. This can be viewed as going against a physician's ethical duty 'to do no harm'" (Vaz et al., 2019).

If CHI research occupies a unique moral status, the extent of its uniqueness has not been examined in depth. This is important because there are many types of CHI research, and the things that make some types of CHI research unique may not hold for all types of CHI research. Notably, Bambery et al. argue explicitly that these features of CHI research generate additional ethical safeguards beyond standard requirements, specifically: (1) a publicly available rationale for the research, (2) independent expert review, (3) protection against community spread of the pathogen, and (4) a system of compensation for harm. Yet Bambery and colleagues argued for this type of extra scrutiny for all CHI research; they did not distinguish between different types of CHI research. What previous discussions of the ethics of CHI research have missed is that distinguishing between CHI models and CHI studies can help clarify what types of CHI research are ethically unique and calibrate when extra ethical attention is needed.

To be fair, I did not realize the importance of this distinction until I was preparing a talk in July 2022 for a panel on CHI research on COVID-19, at the International Association of Bioethics conference in Basel, Switzerland. My role in the panel was to provide a skeptic's view of CHI research done in the United Kingdom during the COVID-19 pandemic. As I discuss further in Chapter 5, as I developed my critique of the UK's CHI research with SARS-CoV-2, I realized that there was a great deal of uncertainty about the value it could offer and the risks to which participants would be exposed, making it difficult to work out whether the research was ethically justified. I began to realize that understanding the difference between models and studies was essential to the ethics of CHI research. I refined my view of this distinction and its ethical importance through conversations with close collaborators (particularly Annette Rid, Frank Miller, and Tom Darton) in a paper considering what virtue ethics can tell us about CHI research that I co-authored with Jeffrey Poomkudy (Poomkudy & Shah, 2024) when consulting with the Indian Council of Medical Research as they were considering guidance for CHI research to be conducted in India for the first time (as discussed in Chapter 6) and while writing this book.

CHI Models Versus Studies

While the distinction between a model and a study is not unique to CHI research, it does play out differently in CHI research than in other scientific endeavors. In general, scientific models are created to increase understanding in some way that is foundational to future research, such as by explaining the relationship between cause and effect. For example, animal models are also often developed prior to human involvement in research to elucidate the mechanisms involved in the condition under study.

In the context of CHI research, developing a controlled human infection *model* has a particular meaning as the necessary first step in a longer process. While animal models are often used prior to CHI research, setting up a model that is safe and reliable in *humans* is critical. Developing a CHI model is a step that directly involves exposing humans to risk. Setting up a CHI model is key for ensuring replicability and safety, and it requires determining the key parameters for future research with this model.

For example, scientists make decisions about the safety of the staff and surrounding community, such as determining the level of biosecurity required for the research facility and deciding what personal protective equipment study staff will use to avoid becoming infected themselves. Researchers have to select and purify the strain of the virus that they will give participants so that they know for certain what they are infecting people with, along with determining the initial dose of the pathogen that will be given to the first person in the study. This includes determining whether to use a weakened version of the pathogen or to use what is circulating in the wild and infecting people—which often involves a trade-off between risk and relevance. Researchers also decide how the dose will be increased if it does not infect enough people at the start. In making these decisions, they must account for the fact that some strains could be much more likely to cause severe symptoms than others. As we saw in Chapter 1, the choice of strain was a consequential decision for Walter Reed's yellow fever studies in Cuba. The decision to use a particularly virulent strain of yellow fever led to three of the four deaths that occurred in that research program (Chaves-Carballo, 2013).

Researchers also select how participants will be infected (e.g., by injection, mosquitoes, pipette). Many, but not all, controlled human malaria infection studies take the approach of placing cups of mosquitos carrying the parasite on the arms of participants until they have had a certain number of bites (Stanisic et al., 2018). By contrast, the UK's model of deliberately infecting people with SARS-CoV-2, the virus that causes COVID-19, used a method that was different from how most people become infected but was designed to reduce the risks to staff members who were infecting participants. They drew up a small amount of the virus into a pipette and then placed the viral particles into participants' nostrils (Jackson et al., 2024). Once participants have been exposed to a pathogen, the research team has to decide how to keep participants safe (e.g., how long to keep them confined, what treatments [if any] to provide, when to intervene with treatment or supportive care, etc.).

After making these decisions, researchers then set out to find what some refer to as the "Goldilocks dose"—an amount of the pathogen needed to infect more than 50% of people without making them too sick (Samuel, 2020). The process of developing a CHI model typically takes between 4 and 12 months. As we will see in Chapter 5, failure to appreciate this distinction and how long creating a model would take led to unjustified hype about CHI research for vaccine testing during the COVID-19 pandemic. Only after the parameters of the CHI model have been set can researchers use the model to conduct CHI *studies* testing interventions like vaccines and treatments.

The difference between models and studies is not just technical, but also has important ethical implications. This distinction matters morally because creating a new model of how to infect people is akin to venturing into the unknown with these participants. Researchers must decide and learn several things before they can establish the development of a reliable and safe way to infect people. For example, once researchers select the strain (or variant) of a pathogen that has a particular level of potency, that strain is used in all subsequent studies with that model. In this way, decisions made during the creation of the model will hold constant in subsequent studies with that model but with more data to support them or understand their implications. As experience grows with using the model safely, CHI studies become much more predictable. This in turn means that CHI studies are generally much less ethically complicated than CHI models. CHI studies rely on previous experience with the model to test new interventions, and they have protocols to follow to make the process controlled and safe. This suggests that, for CHI studies conducted with a model that has already been shown to be safe and reproducible, the ethical issues will not be as complicated as they were for the initial creation of the model. Unless researchers are modifying the model in a significant way, such as by moving the model from a higher-income country where the disease is not circulating to a lower-income country where it is endemic, they can anticipate what will happen and have guidance on how to respond to it.

Admittedly, there might be some exceptions to this general rule. The creation of a new CHI model with a disease that is very well known and characterized, with robust epidemiologic data, might be much simpler than the use of an existing CHI model with a disease that remains poorly understood. Some uncertainty can also be managed by taking a cautious approach—for example, researchers could give the first human participant a dose of the pathogen that is so low it would be considered homeopathic, and escalate doses very gradually, to minimize risk.[1] Nevertheless, it is generally the case that the creation of a new CHI model is more ethically complex and important to scrutinize than the use of an existing model in a CHI study.

Once a CHI model has been developed and shown to be safe, reliable, and reproducible, it can be used in different ways, including to test interventions in CHI studies. For example, a common approach is to give people either an experimental vaccine or a placebo and then

---

[1] I would like to thank Meta Roestenberg and Anna Durbin for this important point.

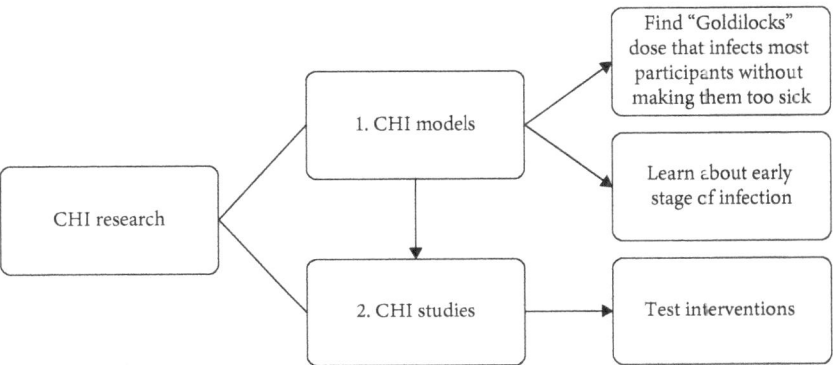

Figure 3.1 Distinction between controlled human infection (CHI) models and studies.

"challenge" them with exposure to a pathogen. If most of the people who got the vaccine stay healthy and people in the placebo group become sick, that provides clear evidence that the vaccine works. CHI studies can also be a good way to test different hypotheses about the immune system. One CHI study, for instance, investigated whether not sleeping enough can make people more susceptible to catching a cold. This study found that people with less than 7 hours of sleep were more likely to be infected with rhinovirus when exposed to it than people who had more than 8 hours of sleep (Cohen et al., 1960/2009). While this finding is intuitive and may not be surprising, it advanced the scientific understanding of sleep and how it relates to the functioning of the immune system. Importantly, the precision of CHI research offers clear advantages over other research, but it also comes with limitations due to the time it takes to set up a model (if one doesn't already exist) and because of its controlled and artificial nature (see Figure 3.1).

Are CHI models or Studies Morally Unique?

With this distinction between models and studies in mind, I now consider the question of whether CHI research is morally unique in depth. I examine several possible reasons that CHI research might be considered morally problematic when compared with other types of research. I conclude that some types of CHI research—such as the creation of a new CHI model or the use of an existing model in a new setting or with a novel population—raise a constellation of ethical issues that are complex and/or not fully resolved by regulations or existing literature and therefore require more caution to carry out. These reasons for extra caution are not present in every type of CHI research, however, nor are they entirely unique to CHI research. Other studies may also occasionally raise the same types of ethical issues. When research raises the same set of unresolved, complex ethical issues as the creation of a new CHI model, however, a similar level of scrutiny may be necessary. In sum, I argue that certain types of CHI research and selected other research can pose several issues that are complex and unresolved, and, until those issues are resolved satisfactorily, additional ethical safeguards are needed.

Is the Social Benefit from CHI Research More Uncertain Than in Other Studies?

Social value is "the importance of the information that a study is likely to produce." (Council for International Organizations of Medical Sciences, 2016). This importance can be based on the information's direct impact on a health problem or from its contribution to deeper understanding of a problem that ultimately can lead to advances. Even negative findings can close out a line of inquiry so that future research can tackle questions more likely to succeed. The social value requirement is the idea that all studies should have sufficient social value to justify their conduct, given that research takes up valuable resources and can expose participants to risk (Wendler & Rid, 2017).

CHI models and CHI studies raise different challenges with respect to measuring their social value. CHI models do not necessarily have considerable value in the short term. In the best-case scenario, a CHI model might yield insights about how diseases can be prevented and/or transmitted. As prime examples of this type of value, consider Walter Reed's yellow fever CHI model and Edward Jenner's proof of concept for smallpox vaccination. Prior to modern scientific understanding of how diseases are transmitted and how to classify viruses to extrapolate transmission methods, CHI research could help fill in the gaps. Most of the time, however, and particularly in the modern era, CHI models are primarily intended to create an approach to deliberate infection that is safe and reproducible and that is to be used for other ends. This means that the primary objective of most CHI models is to find the minimum dose that will infect most people but not make them too sick. This might also lead to other insights, of course, such as which types of people have greater immunity to infection, what happens in the early stages of disease, or how much virus people shed at different stages of infection. However, this is not the kind of value that most would consider to have substantial social value that could justify exposing participants to significant risks (Eyal et al., 2020).

Once a safe, reproducible CHI model has been created, it can be used in future CHI studies that might test treatments or vaccines, or to learn more about the immune response to pathogens. This means that the value of a CHI model can be thought of as encompassing both what is learned in the initial creation of the model and what is gained from the subsequent use of the model in whichever CHI studies are conducted with it. The challenge, then, is that it is impossible to anticipate exactly what these future CHI studies might be. Future uses of the model will depend on many factors, including how much the pathogen is circulating in the world in the future or whether there are good treatment and vaccine candidates to test. This makes the value of a CHI model potentially very high but fundamentally uncertain, in a way that a typical Phase III study is not.

There are other types of research that may also have uncertain social value, although they differ from CHI research in other respects. For example, Phase I trials in healthy volunteers might also have a great deal of uncertainty, given that more than 95% of drugs fail testing and do not go on to market (Dahlin et al., 2016), the amount of potential value for typical Phase I trials in healthy volunteers is not assumed to be very high. It is much more important to assess uncertainty in social value when that value might be high enough to justify significant risk. As discussed in Chapter 5, this is particularly important to address for the use of CHI models in pandemic preparedness or response.

By contrast, assessing the social value of individual CHI studies using an established model is much more like the standard evaluation of the value of research. If a CHI study was designed to provide preliminary efficacy on vaccine candidates and choose the best candidate among a few options to advance for future testing, this has clear value even if it might be more limited. Evaluating the importance of such a study does not require considering the potential value of all subsequent CHI studies with that pathogen. Therefore, running a study with an existing CHI model will generally have less potential value than creating a new CHI model, but what value there is will be clearer.

Although the development of CHI models seems to have uncertain social value in a way that might seem unique, other types of research face similar ethical challenges. As noted above, phase I research can have uncertain social value. Basic science research can be focused on investigating issues that have unclear application in the future and high potential social value depending on what is learned. On the other hand, basic science research typically does not involve exposing human participants to risk. One exception that might prove this rule is *gain of function research*, which involves studying pathogens and determining whether modifying them could result in more deadly pathogens. This research has received extra scrutiny because it could pose risks to third parties, much like CHI research (Selgelid, 2016).

HIV cure (or remission) research, particularly when in the early stages, similarly presented challenges with respect to uncertain social value (Dube et al., 2021). With the availability of highly active antiretroviral therapy, HIV has been transformed from a lethal disease into a chronic condition, and people living with HIV typically have normal lifespans as long as they can remain on therapy. Antiretroviral therapy has side effects, however, and there would be value in eliminating HIV if possible. Many different approaches to eliminating HIV where it hides in the body are being tested, and it seems likely that no single approach will be sufficient to cure someone who is living with HIV (Selgelid, 2016). The only examples of people who have been cured have required receipt of stem cell transplant (Gupta et al., 2019); in those cases, "cure" means that people will no longer live with HIV but will require undergoing a risky procedure that will still require taking medication for the rest of their lives. The value of that type of cure also does not generalize to people who do not otherwise need a stem cell transplant. Thus, the assessment of the value of any given HIV cure research study was highly uncertain, particularly in the early stages of investigating a new approach to achieve remission.

Another example of research with highly uncertain value is that designed to change the minds of policy decision-makers. As an extreme example of this type of research, consider a randomized controlled trial designed to determine whether medication abortion is reversible (Creinin et al., 2020). In this study, participants who were planning to receive a surgical abortion in the future entered the study and received only one of the two drugs needed for medication abortion (mifepristone) and then were randomized to receive (1) progesterone to try to reverse the abortion or (2) placebo. This study was done to try to influence policymakers who were passing legislation requiring clinicians to counsel pregnant people that medication abortion could be reversed. The study planned to enroll 40 patients but had to be stopped after enrolling only 12 patients due to safety concerns. Three patients had severe hemorrhaging that required being taken to the hospital by ambulance.

While the study ultimately involved considerable risks that may be ethically problematic in their own right, for our purposes, the feature of this study that stands out is its uncertain value. When research is aimed at changing the minds of lawmakers, it can be difficult to know what level of evidence will be necessary to do so. It is particularly unclear whether policymakers who are ideologically motivated to pass laws posing barriers to abortion would be likely to be swayed by research demonstrating that it is unsafe or ineffective to try to reverse medication abortion. Thus, the social value of such research is highly uncertain in a way that is similar to the creation of new CHI models but unlike standard research studies.

These examples demonstrate that the development of a new CHI model is not entirely unique in terms of the uncertainty of the potential value, but also shows that CHI research may be helpful in identifying an ethical challenge that extends to some other types of research. In this case, CHI research may serve to demarcate a class of research that requires additional scrutiny because the extra uncertainty regarding the value of research might be hard for standard review processes to notice or evaluate, particularly given the limited guidance available for rigorously assessing social value (Shah, Miller & Darton et al., 2020). This class of research would include CHI models, gain of function research, and research designed to influence ideologically motivated policies; it may also cover other types of research where additional guidance for evaluating social value may be helpful to review committees.

Is CHI Research Different Because Researchers Intend to Make Participants Ill?

As noted above, there is a widespread intuition that CHI research is distinct from other types of research because researchers *intentionally* cause harm to participants by trying to infect them with pathogens. It may be more accurate to say that researchers intend to expose participants to pathogens hoping to find the dose that will infect most of them but not make any of them very ill. This type of intention is somewhat similar to the intent researchers have in other types of trials. For example, in Phase III studies, to test whether vaccines work, researchers randomize participants to receive the vaccine or a placebo injection and wait to determine if the people who got the vaccine are less likely to get infected than the people who received the placebo. While the researchers likely do not relish the prospect of participants getting sick, they foresee that this will happen and, in fact, rely on it for their research to be successful. Indeed, studies anticipate the likely rate of infection so they can be powered to determine whether the vaccine works, and, if the rate of infection is much lower than anticipated, this can be a major problem that would cause a study to stop early due to lack of feasibility.

The fact that researchers in Phase III trials and CHI researchers have a similar intent for their participants to become infected was easy to see during the COVID-19 pandemic. Based on a concern that not enough people would get sick if the trials were not being conducted at a time of active transmission, researchers set up multiple sites and focused enrollment on those that had high rates of transmission of SARS-CoV-2—they were trying to find places where lots of people were getting infected to make sure they had enough participants in their study who were becoming infected. As some scholars explained, "Paradoxically, the number of cases of COVID-19 required to assess vaccine efficacy was rapidly reached given the fact that the pandemic yielded a remarkably high attack rate of disease. This allowed for clear, unassailable conclusions about the vaccine's ability to prevent disease" (Kuter et al., 2021) . An *attack rate* is the number of new cases of the disease divided by the number of people in the population, so this statement is focused on the fact that COVID-19 affected large numbers of people in a short time. Under tremendous pressure to share when results would be available from Phase III trials, Moderna's CEO stated the following: "That first analysis is likely to occur in November, but it's hard to predict exactly which week because it depends on the cases, the number of people getting sick" (Consumer News and Business Channel, 2020). One researcher at a site in Massachusetts even explicitly stated the calculations researchers made to look for places where infection rates were high: "Certain areas in Worcester have had a much higher incidence of COVID infection. . . .We targeted those areas to recruit volunteers" (Spence, 2020).

Admittedly, participants in Phase III vaccine trials conducted during the COVID-19 pandemic may have had a lower chance of becoming infected with SARS-CoV-2 than CHI research participants who were deliberately exposed to the virus. However, this is a difference of degree that is not necessarily as stark as one might think. While CHI researchers intended for most of the participants to become sick, creating a CHI model requires finding a dose of the virus that infects more than half—but not necessarily all—participants. Vaccine researchers typically do not need half of their participants to become infected but they benefit from higher rates of infection than anticipated because that enables them to accrue endpoints faster and produce results that could lead to early authorization or approval of vaccines. Furthermore, Phase III trials also enroll thousands of people, while CHI research typically involves 15–150 people. Some have argued that this makes CHI research ethically preferable to Phase III trials because it "minimizes risk" since fewer people will become sick in CHI research than in a Phase III trial (Su et al., 2021). This suggests that a CHI researcher might intend to infect most of their participants but not a large number of people, while a researcher conducting a Phase III study might need hundreds or even thousands of participants to become infected to show a difference.

Yet there remains a distinction between the intentions of researchers conducting Phase III trials and the intentions of researchers leading CHI studies. While Phase III researchers *foresee* that participants would become infected with a pathogen, CHI researchers *intend* to infect participants with a pathogen. Thus, the intent of CHI researchers to deliberately infect participants with pathogens is a key difference between CHI research and other types of trials. The fact that this distinction exists is important but does not settle the question of whether CHI research is ethically problematic, as will be discussed at the end of the chapter, once we determine all of the ways in which CHI research is ethically unique or unusual.

Is CHI Research Different Because Researchers *Directly* Cause Harm to Participants?

Next, I consider whether CHI research is ethically unique because it requires researchers to directly harm participants. This could be an ethically relevant distinction if it indicates that CHI researchers are more blameworthy than researchers who expose participants to risks in indirect ways, such as researchers who run Phase III trials and wait for participants to become infected in the course of living their lives. First, I demonstrate that there are other studies in which researchers directly expose participants to risk, suggesting that CHI research is not unique in this respect. I then consider whether the distinction between doing versus allowing (or being active vs. passive) provides a basis for viewing challenge studies differently than other studies involving risk.

Other studies are sometimes referred to as "challenge trials" and similarly raise questions about researchers directly causing harm. One interesting example to compare controlled human infection studies to is a "challenge" trial that involves challenging people to an *allergen* rather than a *pathogen*.[2] Previously, the American Academy

---

[2] I would like to thank Divakar Mitthal for this excellent suggestion.

of Pediatrics in the United States recommended avoiding any exposure to potential allergens, like peanuts, during pregnancy and in the first 2 years of life, although these recommendations were withdrawn in 2008 without being replaced with modified guidance (American Academy of Pediatrics, 2000). After learning that infants in Israel were significantly less likely to have peanut allergies than infants in the United Kingdom, and connecting this to the fact that infants in Israel are exposed to peanuts from a very young age through a commonly used snack called Bamba, researchers planned a trial to test whether exposure to peanuts early in life could reduce allergies. The Learning Early about Peanut Allergy (LEAP) trial was an unblinded, randomized controlled trial (Du Toit et al., 2015). Infants who enrolled in the study were considered to be at risk for having peanut allergies, either because they had severe eczema, were allergic to eggs, or both. Infants randomly assigned to the intervention arm received 6 grams of peanut protein each day. This study carried the obvious risk of infants having an allergic reaction to the peanut protein before it was known whether peanut protein exposure would be beneficial to them. The LEAP trial was successful in demonstrating early exposure to peanuts significantly reduces the risk of having a peanut allergy; it reduced the risk by 86% for infants who did not have a reaction to peanuts through a skin test administered at the start of the study, and by 70% in infants who did have a reaction and were assumed to be allergic to peanuts. Nevertheless, examining the ethics of this trial in advance makes it seem more similar than different to CHI studies. In the LEAP trial, as in CHI research, scientists deliberately exposed people to a foreign object that they knew could cause a harmful reaction and immune response in the body, with risks that were significant. Although the LEAP trial offered the prospect of direct benefit if children developed an immune tolerance to the allergen, the same can be true for CHI research involving infections like SARS-CoV-2 that could confer some protection from future infection.

Another type of "challenge" trial that is important to consider is research that provokes symptoms of mental health conditions, which were briefly discussed in Chapter 2 (Miller & Rosenstein, 1997). These studies typically also involve measuring physiological and biochemical changes in the body in response to the challenge. Miller and

Rosenstein have explained that these studies can be used for several purposes, including to help understand the pathophysiology behind the disorders, distinguish between similar but distinct conditions, uncover how available treatments work, help predict treatment response or risk of relapse after stopping therapy, and help develop new diagnostic tests and treatments. For example, psychiatric symptom-provoking studies have been used to establish that panic disorder and obsessive-compulsive disorder (OCD) are different from each other. These uses are analogous to some of the uses of pathogens in infectious challenge studies. Like these categories of uses for psychiatric symptom-provoking studies, infection challenge studies have similarly been used to understand the pathophysiology of SARS-CoV-2, to determine that hepatitis A was distinct from hepatitis B, and to prioritize malaria vaccines and treatments for further study.

Miller and Rosenstein do not suggest that psychiatric symptom-provoking studies are necessarily ethically distinct from other kinds of psychiatric research. They argue that the ethical concerns raised by these studies can be found in other types of nontherapeutic psychiatric research and that the critical ethical issue is that these studies are not being done to benefit the participants but to benefit future patients. One important distinction between psychiatric challenge studies and CHI studies, however, is that psychiatric "challenge" studies could suffer from a therapeutic misconception in which participants think they are receiving care that is for their benefit while researchers are focused on learning information to benefit future patients. Researchers doing symptom-provoking studies typically enroll patients who have not yet started treatment, and these patients may mistake the offer to participate in research with a treatment plan. They may also find the offer of being treated in these studies (after symptoms are provoked, of course) to be a significant inducement that is hard to turn down, particularly if they are finding it difficult to access treatment (Miller & Rosenstein, 1997). Such a concern is much less likely to occur with CHI research—few people would assume that deliberate exposure to a pathogen was intended to benefit them unless they had almost no understanding of the research.

The second ethical issue Miller and Rosenstein raise is about risks and benefits. They note that most symptoms are transient and similar to what these patients commonly experience. However, they provide several examples of patient risks in these types of studies that need to be carefully considered. For example, one patient with OCD said she moved in and out of her house for 3 hours during a severe thunderstorm to check on something in her backyard, reporting that this was both unusual and distressing. To address potential risks, Miller and Rosenstein have several practical suggestions. In addition to independent review to assess the scientific and social value of the study and robust informed consent procedures, they argue for (1) careful development of criteria to exclude people at high risk, including not conducting symptom-provoking challenge studies with people at risk of suicide or those prone to violent behavior; (2) selection of the dose, route of administration, and frequency of administration for the challenge agent to minimize risk (including starting with a less risky approach and slowly escalating); (3) close monitoring of participants that may include isolation or a plan for administering therapy when symptoms become too severe; (4) transparency about the rationale and justification for the study as well as the process of informed consent; and (5) longer-term follow-up of participants, including studies to understand their motivations and any lingering effects of participation. As will be elucidated in the following chapter, these issues and solutions parallel the guidance for CHI research and provide additional reason to believe that CHI research is not ethically unique.

While the existence of other types of "challenge studies" suggests that CHI research is not ethically unique, perhaps all studies that can be called "challenge studies" raise a similar ethical challenge: How can it be ethical for a researcher to directly cause harm to participants? As noted above, this seems intuitively different from the case of a vaccine researcher who waits for participants to become infected while they go about their ordinary lives, both in terms of intent, as argued above, and in how direct the link is between what the researcher does and the risk the participant experiences. The research intervention is what made CHI participants infected with a pathogen, while interactions with others outside of the research study caused participants in Phase III trials to become infected. Yet it is hard to see a difference between the direct imposition of harm in CHI research and any research that involves interventions done for research purposes that can cause harm. It is hard to make a moral distinction between the actions of a researcher who performs a lumbar puncture for research purposes and a CHI researcher who infects a participant with malaria. Thus, the fact that CHI researchers directly cause harm does not seem in any way unique, and is an important issue routinely addressed by review committees in any study that involves non-beneficial procedures done for research purposes only.

Is CHI Research Different Because CHI Researcher Intentionally Cause Net Harm to Participants?

One potential, but ultimately dubious, distinction between CHI research and other studies is that CHI researchers intentionally cause *net* harm to participants by infecting them. Unlike in trials testing new therapies, CHI participants are exposed to risks without the chance of benefit for themselves, but rather to benefit future patients. This idea initially seems promising until one recalls that all nonbeneficial research involves some risk of harm to research participants, as noted above, with the concern that CHI research involves more direct imposition of harm than other studies.

Phase I studies with healthy volunteers involve exposing people to risks of medications that they do not need for their own health but that are being tested for safety in search of medications that can be given to other patients. Even beneficial studies involve procedures that are done purely for research purposes, ranging from surveys to blood draws to lumbar punctures and even liver biopsies. The primary aim of research is not to benefit the participants but to benefit others in the future—and this risk–benefit tradeoff, as noted by Christine Grady and Frank Miller more than 20 years ago (Miller & Grady, 2001)—is not unique to CHI research. In many types of research, researchers may hope that the interventions they are testing are safe and will not harm participants and that nothing will go wrong with the research procedures, but they understand, foresee, and accept that harm might occur to research participants in many different kinds of studies. Ultimately, the ethical concern that deliberate infection is unique because it results in net harm to participants that researchers intend may result from a fundamental confusion between the ethics of clinical research and the ethics of clinical care (Miller, 2004).

Is CHI Research Riskier Than Other Types of Research?

Relatedly, some might argue that CHI research is morally distinct simply because it poses higher risks than other studies. Yet comparing the risks of challenge studies to the risks of other types of research shows that this concern is not borne out by data.

The first question to address is: How risky is CHI research? A systematic review of 284 studies found that the most common CHI research by far involved malaria, influenza, and rhinovirus (a virus that causes common colds) (Adams-Phipps et al., 2023). More than 4,300 participants were enrolled in rhinovirus studies, followed by 3,536 people exposed to influenza viruses, and 1,689 individuals in controlled human malaria infection studies. Notably, however, 33% of these studies did not report any data on adverse events, and 34% did not report any data on serious adverse events (SAEs)—harms that are life-threatening or require hospitalization. The failure to report complications in about one-third of the studies that are in the published literature makes it difficult to know the true level of risk in CHI research. There are also anecdotal reports that are not published but often discussed at meetings with CHI investigators. For instance, one controlled human malaria infection study had a volunteer who left the study before getting treatment and crossed international borders. The study team ultimately contacted Interpol and made sure the participant received treatment. This example was not included in the systematic review, however.

In the two-thirds of studies that reported adverse events, there were 10,325 participants in total. While the study reported a finding that 42–56% of individuals in these studies experienced at least one adverse event, the authors provided more precise ranges across the decades, which showed higher rates of reporting adverse events in the past two decades than had previously occurred. The authors indicate that this is because more studies report adverse events by individual or symptom, rather than just aggregating events over the study.

In studies that quantified adverse events in terms of how severe they were (not including adverse events that are severe enough to be life-threatening or require hospitalization, which will be discussed further below), between 6% and 16% of participants had at least one severe or very severe adverse event. Although only 19 studies included control participants, and only two of those studies reported adverse event data for those in the control arm, there were adverse events reported in the control arm—between 10% and 17% of participants in control arms reported at least one adverse event. Some CHI researchers recount that it is extremely important to include control arms for studies of pathogens that cause symptoms that are routinely experienced by people in daily life, noting that people routinely have unexplained headaches, body aches, and even fevers that they may not have even noticed if they weren't asked to record their symptoms carefully.

Of the 65% of studies that reported SAEs that could cause death or result in an individual being hospitalized, only 23 out of 10,016 people, or 0.2% of participants, had at least one SAE. For example, Norovirus CHI studies, which were the studies that had the most SAEs per participant challenged, reported severe vomiting and diarrhea as an SAE (Bernstein et al., 2015). *Plasmodium* CHI research had the most reported SAEs overall, and these included a probable case of acute myocarditis where the participant had a normal cardiac magnetic resonance imaging (MRI) study after about 5 months, when the issue had mostly resolved (Bastiaens et al., 2016). There were other studies that involved challenging people with pathogens more than once, and one additional person had at least one severe adverse event, but no deaths were reported. These adverse events included diarrhea and vomiting from *E. coli* infection or Norovirus that were severe enough to require intravenous fluid or oral medication, and dilated cardiomyopathy (a disease of the heart muscle that makes it harder to pump blood around the body) that could have been related to being infected with influenza B. While none of the studies reported long-term complications that failed to resolve with time and treatment, some studies did not explain if or when the issue resolved.

Finally, it is interesting that more than 90% of the studies (286/308) described the steps they took to minimize risk. Participants were screened, which included questions about their medical histories, to ensure that they were not at elevated risk from the pathogen. For example, participants were asked about the potential for pregnancy and birth control requirements. Participants were also often excluded from studies if they worked in occupations that could lead them to spread the pathogen to others at risk, such as excluding people who had jobs in the food service industry from a CHI with *Salmonella*.

Other reviews have also found that SAEs are rare in CHI research. CHI studies with malaria have typically been done with *Plasmodium falciparum* with an impressive safety record. However, one study with *P. vivax* inadvertently uncovered a genetic polymorphism that appears to have limited the bioavailability of the drug primaquine, which was administered to cure malaria, when two participants had multiple relapses of malaria (Bennett et al., 2013). Relapses have not been found in subsequent studies, however (Bennett et al., 2016).

CHI research has frequently been compared to Phase 1 studies with healthy volunteers (Walker et al., 2022), which similarly expose participants to net risks—risks that are not offset by the chance for participant benefit. There is a considerable amount of research on the risks involved in Phase I trials with healthy volunteers that is helpful to compare to the data on CHI research (Fisher et al., 2018; Johnson et al., 2016; McManus et al., 2019; Walker & Fisher, 2019). One systematic review of 475 phase I trials with more than 27,000 participants found that there were no SAEs reported in these trials and low rates of mild-moderate adverse events, although the authors raised the possibility that adverse events are underreported. More specifically, the authors found that "The rate of mild and moderate adverse events was a median of 1147.19 per 1000 participants (interquartile range, 651.52–1730.9) and 46.07 per 1000 participants/AE monitoring day (interquartile range, 17.80–77.19)" (Johnson et al., 2016).

These data, although incomplete, are consistent with suggesting that CHI research, in general, is comparable to but may be somewhat more risky than other research. Mild adverse events are common in both types of research, but moderate and severe adverse events were more likely to be reported in CHI research than in Phase I studies. Notably, however, CHI research has reported low rates of SAEs and no deaths. Only rarely have these harms been long-lasting. CHI studies with malaria tend to report a much lower rate of harm, suggesting that the use of established models may be comparable to Phase I studies. This suggests that CHI research may sometimes be riskier than other types of research but is not always or generally more risky—it simply depends on the type of research being done. Thus, available data on risks have some important limitations but do not suggest that CHI research is ethically distinct from other types of research in this respect.

Does CHI Research Uniquely Exceed the Upper Limit of Allowable Risk in Research?

While the previous discussion suggests that CHI research does not pose higher levels of risk than other types of research, it is interesting to note that influential international ethical guidance uses CHI research as an example of research that might exceed the upper limit of risk that should be permitted in research. The World Health Organization's Council for International Organizations for the Medical Sciences (CIOMS) does not explicitly state what the upper limit of risk should be. This is consistent with a long history of broad (but not complete) agreement in the literature that there should be an upper limit of risk in research, even though it is very difficult to specify what that limit should be. Rather than setting a limit, CIOMS guidance uses two intuitively plausible examples of what would exceed the threshold of permissible risk—the examples of CHI models with anthrax and Ebola virus disease (assuming the current state of affairs in which there are no good ways to treat these diseases).

These examples are useful to generate intuitions about the upper limit of risk; almost anyone can understand them and have a sense of whether they think permitting this type of research would be right or wrong. Yet it is also possible that these examples could be misleading The intuitive "yuck reaction" discussed in Chapter 2 may drive some of the intuition that such studies should not be conducted. The fear and disgust associated with diseases like Ebola virus disease and anthrax may be triggered by these examples and serve as confounders, making our intuitions less reliable.

Perhaps more importantly, the level of risk in these studies appears to far exceed CHI models and CHI studies that have been conducted in the modern era. There is a high level of risk involved in exposing participants to a potentially lethal disease where existing treatments have limited efficacy. To this point, no researchers, to my knowledge, have proposed developing CHI models for these pathogens. Even if there were such proposals, the risk level involved would depend on many factors. There are different ways to conduct CHI research that could make any given study much less risky than the experience of infection from a circulating virus. This suggests that, depending on how a CHI study is designed, even these examples could involve much lower risk than anticipated by the authors of the CIOMS guidelines. For example, CHI research with tuberculosis uses the BCG vaccine as the route of exposure. Dengue CHI research similarly uses a failed vaccine candidate to induce infection. For CHI research, the key issue is not necessarily what the disease is as understood and experienced by the general public, but rather which strain is selected and whether there is a way to infect people that is controlled and unlikely to cause lasting harm. This suggests that, in theory at least, there could be a way to design a relatively low-risk CHI model even for diseases that would normally have a high fatality rate, depending on whether a strain could be identified that would not pose any risk of long-term harm or death.

Thus, despite the way it is portrayed in prominent ethical guidance, CHI research does not necessarily exceed the upper limit of risk. As with other research, the risk level simply depends on the details of the particular trial.

Is CHI Research Different Because It Alone Poses Risks to Third Parties?

Another important difference between CHI research and other types of studies was suggested by Bambery and colleagues in 2015. These scholars noted that CHI research may pose risks to people who did not enroll in studies themselves or give their consent to be exposed to pathogens—sometimes referred to as "bystanders" or "third parties." Risks to third parties can loom even larger when the pathogen being studied is not circulating in the region, as was the case with a Zika virus CHI model that was being contemplated in Baltimore. This raises the concern that an ordinary member of the community would not otherwise be on notice of the risk of being infected with that pathogen and may not know to take precautions.

Third-party risks are challenging because there is limited guidance in the regulations and bioethics literature about how to manage these risks, so management of these risks can be a bit like flying blind. In the case of the Zika virus CHI, one Institutional Review Board (IRB) member raised the question about third-party risks but was informed that this was not an issue. A subsequent ethics panel chaired by this author paused the study for this concern (along with the concern that the trial did not have compelling social value given other research that was taking place) (Shah et al., 2018), as discussed in Chapter 5. In March 2022, the Secretary's Advisory Committee on Human Research Protections (SACHRP) issued guidance on The Protection of Non-Subjects from Research Harm. This guidance makes clear that IRBs do have a responsibility to identify and minimize risk to third parties, or non-participants, but advises IRBs not to routinely review these risks unless the level of risk to non-participants is more than minimal (Secretary's Advisory Committee on Human Research Protections, 2022). How IRBs should address these and determine when the level of risk to non-participants is acceptable is left unclear, however: "SACHRP recommends that IRBs consider the need to formalize in policy the review of risk to non-subjects and the referral to or coordination of review with other expert external or institutional bodies and functions."

Yet CHI research is not the only type of research to raise concerns about third-party risk. HIV cure studies involve taking participants who are well-controlled on antiretrovirals off of their medication to try and lure the virus out of hiding and find ways to eliminate it from the body. In these HIV cure studies, participants may experience viral rebound and become much more likely to transmit HIV, where they were not before. Thus, these studies pose risks of infecting third parties, specifically the sexual partners of trial participants. This is just one example of a type of research where a participant's involvement could lead to risks for third parties. People enrolled in research involving wearable devices that they take into their daily lives may expose members of their households to risks of privacy loss or even of being reported to authorities if their behavior raises concerns about abuse or neglect. Some studies of radioactive therapies to treat cancer can expose family members to radioactivity that continues to emanate from the research participant. This suggests that although CHI research is not ethically unique by virtue of raising risks to third parties, the fact that CHI research raises risks to third parties places it in a special class. Researchers conducting studies that expose people to third-party risks operate in territory that is lightly regulated, if at all. The limited regulatory guidance suggests that greater caution and attention to the resulting ethical issues may be necessary for this third aspect of CHI research that makes it ethically unusual.

Is CHI Research Different Because It Places Limitations on the Right to Withdraw?

When CHI research has the potential to expose third parties to risk, a strategy that researchers use to manage this risk is to confine participants when they are infectious. This common approach puts pressure on the right to withdraw from research: if participants were to leave the study early, they could expose others to risk. The right to withdraw is widely considered an important protection for research participants. Many international regulations and ethical guidelines emphasize the importance of voluntary participation in research that includes protecting the right to withdraw (Brazil National Council of Health, 2012; Council of Europe, 2005; Council for International Organizations of Medical Sciences, 2016; World Medical Association, 2013). For instance, the US Federal Regulations provide as follows, "In seeking informed consent investigators must provide each subject with a statement that participation is voluntary, refusal to participate will involve no penalty or loss of benefits to which the subject is otherwise entitled, and the subject may discontinue participation at any time without penalty or loss of benefits to which the subject is otherwise entitled" (Office for Human Research Protection, 2018). Although this requirement appears to place stringent requirements on investigators, the interpretation of this language by the Office for Human Research Protections makes clear that it may not be strictly necessary to allow participants to withdraw at any time, no questions asked. For instance, researchers are advised to speak with participants to understand their wishes because a participant who decides to withdraw might be interested in leaving one part of the study but fine with continued participation in another (or with continued use of their data) (Office for Human Research Protections, 2010).

While some ethicists have argued that it could be ethically justifiable to waive the right to withdraw in some cases (Chwang, 2008), this is a minority view and one that is not consistent with existing regulations. Furthermore, Schafer and Wertheimer have forcefully defended the right to withdraw from an ethical perspective, identifying several reasons for the general ethical rule allowing participants to withdraw at any time (Schaefer & Wertheimer, 2010). These reasons include the information asymmetry between researchers and participants, the inability of research participants to hedge on their decisions, the uncertainty inherent in research, the degree of bodily invasion that can occur in research, and the need to support public trust in research. Thus, there is widespread agreement that the right to withdraw should be respected. In that light, CHI research may seem to be ethically unique because restrictions on the right to withdraw might be important to protect both participants and third parties.

Notably, there are other examples of studies in which withdrawing from research early can be risky for participants or others. For example, oncology trials that require using chemotherapy to ablate the immune system before transplantation leave participants very vulnerable to infection. If they were to leave the hospital when their immune systems were not functioning, this would be very risky. In those trials, participants are still allowed to withdraw from research, but advised not to leave the hospital until their immune system recovers. As discussed above, if a participant were to withdraw early from an HIV cure study that involves closely monitored treatment interruptions, they might have an undetectable viral load at the time they leave the study. When the virus begins to rebound, these participants could unknowingly expose others to the risk of HIV infection. Studies testing the effects of sleep deprivation by randomizing participants to conditions of partial or total sleep deprivation often require confinement for a period of time (Williams et al., 2024). In such a study, it may be possible that participants who leave the study early and decide to drive home or return to work could find that a lack of sleep could disrupt their performance and put them and others at risk. Thus, while it may not be routine in research that early withdrawal poses risks to non-participants, CHI research is hardly unique in this way.

Additionally, the concern that CHI researchers might place restrictions on the right to withdraw in light of these risks is largely unfounded. Holly Lynch has pointed out that although researchers can take steps to avoid withdrawal, such as enhanced informed consent processes so participants really understand what they are getting into or providing clear reasons for the safeguards being used, researchers lack legal authority to keep unwilling participants in isolation (Fernandez Lynch, 2020). In other words, if a research participant decides to leave a research facility, researchers cannot force them to stay. Researchers could take certain steps to minimize risk. For example, Miller and Grady have noted that "Whereas subjects may not be allowed to leave the research facility for a specified period, this does not preclude their right to withdraw from further exposure to infectious agents and/or other unwanted procedures" (Miller & Grady, 2001). Researchers could offer to discontinue all research procedures and stop data collection but still ask participants to remain in confinement until they are no longer infectious.

Yet the fact remains that researchers rarely if ever have the authority to prevent participants from leaving a research facility. To the extent an informed consent document is a contract (which is not entirely legally clear), the law generally disfavors compelling someone to hold up their end of the bargain. Rather than requiring "specific performance" of what someone agreed to do initially, the legal remedy for not upholding an agreement is usually to pay damages to the person who was harmed. Because the power of the state would be needed to coerce people to remain in isolation, public health law can provide legal authority to require participants to remain confined in some cases. Public health laws can compel people to isolate for some diseases, like tuberculosis, that are present in a given area. However, public health laws do not typically require isolation or quarantine for very common diseases that can be risky, such as influenza. Furthermore, governments usually do not have reasons to pass laws to require quarantine or isolation for diseases that are not common. This means that some CHI research on diseases that are not widely circulating, such as a Zika CHI model in Baltimore, would likely not be able to rely on existing laws to compel participants to isolate from others in the community.

Thus, the limitations on the right to withdraw posed in CHI research are not usually absolute and are similar to restrictions placed on participants in other studies. To the extent they go beyond other research, they are justified by laws created to protect the public's health—not by research ethics or regulations. When researchers are able to draw on existing laws to report participants and require them to take public health precautions, the fact that this CHI research straddles the line between research and public health may be unique, but this will not be true for all or even most CHI research. As noted above, the majority of CHI studies involve malaria or viruses that cause the common cold, neither of which are subject to public health laws that require isolation or confinement.

What are the implications for CHI research? While most issues related to the right to withdraw from CHI research can be dealt with in the same manner that they are dealt with elsewhere, one interesting suggestion Lynch makes that may require a different approach for CHI research is the idea that if withdrawal from research would be unacceptably risky, that research should not be conducted in the first place. For example, if a participant leaving the study early could potentially cause a global pandemic and researchers would have no legal authority to stop them, this might be a reason not to conduct a CHI study. This possibility suggests that, instead of being concerned that CHI research could place extra limitations on the right to withdraw, it might be better to focus on the opposite problem: there may be times when the need to respect the right to withdraw means that it is ethically problematic to conduct CHI research. CHI research might therefore be unique in the sense that it could be ethically unacceptable if withdrawal is unacceptably risky, and this ethical issue should be assessed in advance by researchers and review committees, as will be addressed in Chapter 4's framework.

Is CHI Research Different Because It Pays More Than Other Research?

There is a common perception that CHI research participation can be very lucrative. The close monitoring that usually occurs in CHI research can involve periods of confinement and an intense schedule of study visits, leading to relatively high payments for research participation. Perhaps the longest period of confinement for a CHI was 29 days. Many CHI research requires that participants come back to the clinic site every day for a month or longer. Thus, even if participants are paid a minimum wage for their time, the total amount of compensation can be substantial. One survey of CHI investigators found very variable amounts of payment, however, ranging from nothing to £3393 (or approximately US$4,322 with current exchange rates) (Grimwade et al., 2020). CHI models with SARS-CoV-2 paid participants above this range; participants could earn up to £4,470 (approximately US$5600) (Oxford Vaccine Group, 2020).

Although these payments seem high compared to the small amounts that participants might be paid for survey research or other short-term studies, they are in line with—or even less than—what healthy people who enroll in Phase I studies can make. Jill Fisher and colleagues conducted a study of healthy volunteers who screened for more than 1,000 trials at 73 sites over the course of 3 years (Fisher et al., 2021). They found that participants were paid an average of US$3070, with a range of US$150–13,000. Anecdotally, some CHI researchers report difficulty in recruiting participants because they cannot compete with how much participants could earn in Phase I trials.

A more complete analysis of the ethics of payments in CHI research will be conducted in Chapter 4. For present purposes, it is important to determine whether there is anything ethically unique about CHI research with respect to payment. Although CHI research tends to pay less than Phase I research, perhaps it exacerbates existing concerns related to monetary motivations. One concern that arises with participants in Phase I trials is that they may become repeat participants, or "guinea pigs," to earn money. Yet the available evidence suggests that many people who enroll in CHI research do not necessarily have prior research experience and typically are not enrolling in more than one study at a time (Kraft et al., 2019; Marsh et al., 2022).

Another worry is that CHI participants may be so motivated by money that they are not carefully weighing the risks involved. The concern over monetary motivations has led some to raise concerns of coercion and undue inducement. *Coercion* involves a threat to take away something that a person is entitled to have, while *undue inducement* is the worry that participants will be so blinded by the money that they will fail to perceive the risks and compromise their values (Largent & Fernandez Lynch, 2017). As Alan Wertheimer and Frank Miller have argued, concerns about coercion are entirely misplaced because an offer to pay someone to participate in research does not force them to do it but rather expands their options (Wertheimer & Miller, 2014).

As will be discussed further in Chapter 4, the available data suggest that worries about undue inducement are also misplaced. Data suggest that CHI participants do not have a higher tolerance for risks compared to the general population, except perhaps a greater willingness to take on risk for the benefit of others (Hoogerwerf et al., 2020). Furthermore, like participants in other trials (Stunkel & Grady, 2011), participants in CHI research may have some monetary motivations, but they are rarely solely focused on the money. Rather, their motivations tend to be mixed, involving not only a desire for monetary incentives but also altruism, interest in science, curiosity, or even an interest in having new experiences (Kraft et al., 2019; Oguti et al., 2019).

Finally, there is no clear evidence that CHI participants are uniquely compromising fundamental values or interests for the sake of earning money. In a qualitative study of CHI malaria participants, we probed to understand whether participation was inconsistent with their values and preferences, but we could not find any indication that this was occurring. One participant said that being engaged in the study required taking medicine, and he generally tried to avoid taking any kind of medications or drugs in his everyday life. When pressed on why he chose to enroll in the study, he indicated that this was a general practice, but not an absolute prohibition, and he thought it was worthwhile to participate in the study even if it meant that he had to take medication (S. A. Kraft et al., 2019). Although there might be cases where participants who are altruistically motivated are taken advantage of in CHI research, or where participants compromise their deeply held values and preferences for the money, there is no solid evidence that this occurs in CHI research, and it seems unlikely that it occurs in CHI research to a greater degree than in other studies.

Implications of the Moral Distinction Between CHI Research and Other Types of Research

The above analysis suggests that CHI research is unusual in that it raises five ethical issues that are complex and/or not fully resolved: (1) uncertain social value, (2) researchers intend to expose participants to diseases, (3) participants face uncertain and potentially high risk, (4) third parties can be put at risk, and (5) early withdrawal can pose risks to participants or others outside the study. CHI models require extra scrutiny because they have highly uncertain social value and risk, and they also set the parameters for future CHI studies regarding the ethical issues raised by these trials. Importantly, however, CHI research is not necessarily more risky or more lucrative than other types of research. The issues raised by CHI research that are unusual do require extra attention, particularly in the face of limited regulatory guidance, and they motivate the need for an ethical framework for CHI research that will be laid out in the next chapter.

Conclusion

CHI research can be distinct from other types of research because it can raise five complex, unresolved ethical issues at once: (1) CHI models have a great deal of uncertainty about their value, (2) researchers intend to expose participants to illness, (3) the risks to participants can be uncertain and high, (4) third parties may be exposed to risk, and (5) in some cases, withdrawal from CHI research may be risky for participants or third parties. Not all of these features arise in all CHI research. However, when a new CHI model is being created, there is high uncertainty or novelty, and these questions are grappled with in particular ways that then set the parameters for future CHI studies. What is needed, then, is an ethical framework specially designed to extend the capacity of our existing research ethics oversight systems to better calibrate the scrutiny CHI research receives. In the next chapter, I will provide just that.

4

Ethical Guidance and Frameworks for CHI Models and Studies

Q: What was your first reaction to the idea of a COVID-19 infection study?
A: It seems like it may have ethical issues, but I'm not in charge of that.
    —Prospective volunteer for COVID-19 CHI research

For most of the history of controlled human infection (CHI) research, ethics lagged behind science (to the extent it was considered at all). For instance, several years after the Willowbrook Hepatitis C studies were conducted in the 1950s, they were initially critiqued by Henry Beecher (Beecher, 1966), and ultimately the subject of a debate in the literature about whether they were ethical (Goldby, 1971; Krugman, 1971). Although CHI research continued into the modern era and accelerated in the 1990s (Roestenberg et al., 2018), the first sustained ethical treatment of CHI research was written in 2001 (Miller & Grady, 2001). Only a handful of articles about CHI research ethics were written after this piece (Bambery et al., 2016; Hope & McMillan, 2004; Shah et al., 2018). When CHI research began being considered for COVID-19, however, the examination of ethical issues exploded. In particular, when the COVID-19 pandemic hit, it inspired a dramatic increase in ethical analysis of CHI research. From 2020 to 2021, more than 100 papers were written about the ethics of CHI studies to address COVID-19—which means that there were more papers on CHI research ethics in the first 2 years of the pandemic than ever before (Katzer et al., 2023). The World Health Organization (WHO) quickly mobilized a group of experts to address the ethics of CHI research and released three guidance documents, with one more in development (WHO Working Group, 2020; World Health Organization [WHO],

Intentionally Infecting Humans. Seema K. Shah, Oxford University Press. © Seema K. Shah 2026.
DOI: 10.1093/9780197667927.003.0004

2022, 2024). In December 2023, the Indian Council of Medical Research published the first country-specific guidance for conducting CHI research (Indian Council of Medical Research, 2023). While the increase in research on the topic and the availability of international guidance documents has advanced the conversation substantially, certain aspects of the ethics of CHI research remain overlooked.

One major limitation of this literature (including my own contributions) was the failure to recognize the ethically relevant distinction between creating a new CHI model versus using an established model in a CHI study, as noted in the previous chapter. Importantly, a CHI model should be understood as the first step in a longer process, depending on how it might be used in future CHI studies (Samuel, 2021). As I show further below, while the initial need to create a CHI model has been recognized to some degree, particularly with respect to the time it takes and some of the steps involved, the ethical relevance of this fact has not been given sufficient attention.

As explained in Chapter 3, developing a new model requires venturing into the many unknowns about a pathogen and is a process that often reveals the limits of existing knowledge. It raises many complex and/or unresolved ethical issues and sets the parameters for future CHI studies with that model. Once key decisions are made for a CHI model, they are set in place for subsequent studies with the same model. This means that certain aspects of the ethics of subsequent studies with that model are already determined once the model has been created. Ethical analysis of future studies with a model can benefit from previous work, as they can rely on evidence from the model and focus on whether and how the study deviates from the model.

Notably, there are some exceptions to this general rule. The research process will not necessarily be linear, and some CHI studies will remain riskier than others. For instance, CHI malaria and cholera studies involve illnesses that can be successfully treated with specific treatments or supportive care, whereas CHI studies with dengue or influenza carry higher risk that cannot be fully ameliorated with existing therapies. The ethical issues involved in interpreting evidence from prior research and evaluating risks are not unlike the issues presented by other types of research, however. Additionally, some models might be able to rely on substantial epidemiological data about diseases that have been circulating for a long time and are well understood, while others will involve diseases that are poorly understood because they are newly emerging or have long been neglected. This suggests that there may be some models that pose less uncertainty than others, and applying this framework will require some exercise of judgment about when to dial up the scrutiny and when to dial it down. Nevertheless, one key insight of this chapter is that for CHI studies conducted with a model that has already been shown to be safe and reproducible, the ethical issues will be less complex and *extra ethical scrutiny is generally not necessary.*

Following on the insight in Chapter 3 that CHI research raises a set of complex and/or unresolved ethical issues, this chapter provides a framework for conducting this complex research ethically. I first review existing ethics literature and guidance for CHI research and demonstrate that there has not been enough attention to the distinction between CHI models and CHI studies, and the moral implications of that distinction been made clearly enough (Bambery et al., 2016; Hope & McMillan, 2004; Miller & Grady, 2001; Shah et al., 2018). To provide a framework that incorporates distinction, I draw upon a few main sources that I will first review: ethical guidance from the WHO; a published ethical framework I have co-authored with an international, multidisciplinary group (Shah, Miller & Darton et al., 2020); and application of this ethical framework and the WHO guidance to the creation of a Hepatitis C virus (HCV) CHI model (Rid et al., 2023). I then provide a consolidated ethical framework that brings together important insights from existing guidance and clearly delineates considerations as they apply to CHI models *and* CHI studies to provide ethical criteria for justifying and conducting CHI research.

Notably, these frameworks are largely consistent with a foundational and influential ethical framework for clinical research (Emanuel et al., 2000, 2004), with some adaptations for the aspects of CHI research that are unusual. In particular, certain benchmarks have been combined (i.e., social value and scientific validity), and some have been renamed to specify what is required or broaden what they contain (e.g., collaborative partnership is referred to as engagement with relevant parties). Two criteria have been added due to their salience in CHI research (i.e., suitable site selection and proportionate payment).

The fact that existing guidelines specific to CHI research build on an existing and more general research ethics framework lends them deeper conceptual grounding; it also may make it easier for ethics reviewers to integrate ethical considerations for CHI research into their practice.

Finally, I acknowledge some exceptions to the general rule that CHI models require extra ethical attention and specialized review in terms of models that not might need extra scrutiny as well as studies that might require it (e.g., use of a CHI model with a population that is very different from the groups that have already been involved in testing, such as people living in low- and middle-income countries with preexisting immunity and immunocompromised people). These insights will lead to an analysis of the ongoing expansion of CHI research in Chapter 6, where I will focus on the use of CHI research in newer populations.

Ethics Literature

In the existing ethics literature on CHI research, the ethical distinction between creating a new CHI model versus using an established model in a CHI study has not received sufficient attention. In 2001, Miller and Grady provided a clear description of the need to develop challenge models before they could be used in challenge studies to test vaccines and treatments (2001). They also delineated a spectrum of risk for candidate diseases for human challenge models, concluding that there may be some types of pathogens that would be too risky to use in a challenge model. However, when they argued that there was nothing ethically unique about this type of research and provided a helpful set of questions to identify the ethical issues that might arise, they focused on the use of an established challenge model in a study— and not on the creation of the model in the first instance. A few years later, Hope and McMillan built on this work and similarly focused their ethical attention on the use of CHI studies and not on CHI models. The examples they chose to discuss reflected the dichotomy between models and studies in an interesting way. Hope and McMillan discussed historical examples of challenge *models* but contemporary examples of challenge *studies*, such as studies with malaria, cholera, influenza, and pneumococcus (2004). This may have led them to draw a contrast between riskier and more ethically questionable research in the past and less risky and problematic research in the modern era.

In 2015, Bambery and colleagues made a quick but important ethical distinction between CHI models and CHI studies that is easy to miss without a close reading of their text. Throughout their article, they used the terms "challenge study" and "challenge model" interchangeably (Bambery et al., 2016). Like Hope and McMillan, they also provided an ethical analysis of two different examples of CHI research that focused on historical challenge models but modern-day CHI studies. The first was Edward Jenner's inoculation of James Phipps with cowpox followed by a smallpox challenge, which we discussed in the Introduction as one of the earliest examples of a challenge study. Recall that, in Chapter 1, we distinguished between historical "challenge studies" that were not subject to the same protections and oversight of modern research and that typically were characterized by practices that would now be criticized as ethically problematic. The second example Bambery and colleagues used was described as more "contemporary" and involved the use of established CHI models with malaria in a CHI study testing vaccines. These examples are different from each other in many ways, and the authors highlighted some of them—in particular, they noted the increased risk and potential for benefit in Jenner's model, along with a lack of consent (Bambery et al., 2016). However, they did not discuss the ethical distinction between these two examples by recognizing that one involved creating a new CHI model and the other involved the use of an established CHI model in a study.

Yet there was one place in the paper where Bambery and colleagues did distinguish between models and studies. In a table that lays out specific criteria for challenge studies, they required four protections above and beyond standard review: (1) independent review, (2) publicly available rationale, (3) protection of public, and (4) compensation for harm. In this table (but not in the paper), they place additional requirements on the creation of a new challenge model. For challenge studies, they indicated that the independent review requirement entails approval by a research ethics committee and by the Food and

Drug Administration in the United States. Yet they suggest that additional scrutiny is needed for the creation of a new model by posing the following question: "If the study involves a new challenge model, has it been reviewed and approved by two independent experts in infectious diseases?" (Bambery et al., 2016). Whether this approach to independent review is the right one for the creation of new challenge models is debatable, but Bambery and colleagues were astute to mark this difference and apply an additional procedural protection to the creation of CHI models. As we discuss further below, there are additional ethical differences between models and studies that should be included in an ethical framework for CHI research.

In the subsequent explosion of articles on CHI ethics during the COVID-19 pandemic, many ethicists failed to distinguish between CHI models and CHI studies in a way that had both ethical and practical significance for the success of their arguments. In Chapter 5, I will evaluate the arguments made for and against using CHI research on SARS-CoV-2 during the COVID-19 pandemic in greater depth; in this chapter, I zoom in to examine the issues that arose because many ethicists (including myself) did not realize the ethical importance of the scientific distinction between developing a model and using an established model in a study.

Much of the ethics literature on the use of CHI research to address COVID-19 did not appreciate the need to create a CHI model before that model could be used to test interventions like vaccines. Many ethicists directly contrasted CHI research with Phase III vaccine research to argue that testing vaccines in CHI studies would be faster than conducting "traditional vaccine trials." For instance, Schaefer and colleagues argued: "In traditional vaccine trials, . . . large trials with substantial follow-up time to accumulate enough cases are needed to test vaccine efficacy. A challenge study guarantees uniform exposure, so potentially can be done faster and with fewer participants. This approach could speed up vaccine development by eliminating ineffective candidates early on and accelerating field trials of the most promising vaccines" (Schaefer et al., 2020). Several ethics articles about CHI research during the COVID-19 pandemic, including one I co-authored, focused on the use of CHI studies to learn more about the early stages of disease or test vaccines and treatments without giving specific ethical consideration to the initial step of creating a CHI model (Calina et al., 2020; Holm, 2020; Jamrozik & Selgelid, 2020; Lucido, 2020; McPartlin et al., 2020; Schaefer et al., 2020; Shah, Miller & Darton et al., 2020).

This failure to recognize the need to create a model before using it to test vaccines distorted consideration of the social value of the initial research as well as its risks and benefits. For example, in a paper examining the issue of whether CHI research on COVID-19 could undermine public trust, Nir Eyal introduces the fact that the United Kingdom has conducted what he refers to as "COVID-19 human challenge trials." He then explains, "In standard COVID-19 vaccine HCTs, consenting adult volunteers are randomised to receive either that vaccine at the dose and regimen being investigated, or contro." (Eyal, 2024). Yet in the initial UK CHI research that Eyal was contemplating in this article, investigators were developing a model and exposed all participants to the March 2020 strain (SARS-CoV-2/human/GBR/484861/2020) of the virus. Eighteen of the 34 volunteers were infected in the final analysis, none of whom received a vaccine (Killingley et al., 2022).

Some ethics articles did consider the need to create a model but underestimated the length of that process, along with its ethical complexity. This ethical analysis also typically considered the ethics of developing a model and using it to test vaccines as one value proposition, rather than two separate research protocols that would each need to be evaluated separately. In perhaps the earliest article on the potential use of CHI research in the COVID-19 pandemic, Eyal, Lipsitch, and Smith argued that human challenge studies could accelerate licensure of a COVID-19 vaccine while acknowledging that a "controlled challenge model" would first need to be standardized before it could be used to test vaccines. They estimated that the process of developing a CHI model "may take several weeks" (Eyal et al., 2020). By contrast, an article by Deming and some colleagues, none of whom is an ethicist, estimated that the creation of a robust CHI model could take 1–2 years and would not be able to speed up vaccine development (2020).

By fall of 2020, there was increasing recognition among ethicists that "traditional vaccine trials" were moving more quickly than anticipated and that CHI research would take longer than many had surmised.

I co-authored a paper led by Christine Grady that explicitly recognized the time it could take to create a model and the rapid pace with which vaccines were being tested. In August 2020, we concluded that the ethical tradeoffs favored more traditional vaccine research over CHI research to accelerate vaccine development (2020). In November, based on the estimate by Deming and colleagues about how long it would take to develop a CHI model (along with concerns about the risks involved to participants and to public trust), some ethicists went further to argue that the development of a CHI model with SARS-CoV-2 would be unethical (Kahn et al., 2020). Finally, in December 2020, Spinola and colleagues focused on the ethical challenges of developing a CHI model, noting that the risks involved would depend on the dose and strain of virus. Importantly, this group emphasized the uncertainty involved in creating a model and selecting strains and doses but focused more on the potential risks than the time it might take to develop the model (Spinola et al., 2020).

As will be discussed in Chapter 5, while concerns about risks in the creation of a CHI model with SARS-CoV-2 were not necessarily borne out due to the very cautious approach to dosing taken by researchers in the United Kingdom, those who predicted limited utility from CHI research given the time it would take to develop a model were on target. The creation of the first CHI model with SARS-CoV-2 took approximately 1 year (Killingley et al., 2022), and subsequent models had to be created with different strains as the virus continued to evolve; these CHI models were therefore too slow to be able to accelerate initial vaccine development.

Finally, there has been more recent attention to the creation of new models with other pathogens, and for HCV in particular. Annette Rid and colleagues have published an analysis of the ethics of creating a new CHI model with HCV and focused their attention on the ethical issues that arise when creating a model (2023). They provide 10 ethical considerations, drawing from previous literature and WHO guidance, and note that their analysis can help guide future studies with the model but with slightly different implications. Specifically, they note that social value and the risk–benefit ratio will be more narrowly focused on the specific research questions that could be addressed in future CHI studies using the model.

It is unclear why the ethics literature has not fully recognized the importance of distinguishing CHI models from CHI studies. It could be that the early literature focused on the use of established models in CHI studies at a time when new models were not being created as frequently. Additionally, ethicists who wrote about CHI research during the COVID-19 pandemic were focused on the creation of a model with an emerging infectious disease, which had two layers of uncertainty because so little was known about COVID-19 and researchers were also looking to create a new model. Ethicists may therefore have assumed the most important uncertainty was connected to the unknowns about SARS-CoV-2. Furthermore, because the articles that have addressed the distinction typically have also included scientists or CHI researchers as authors, another possibility is that ethicists writing without this kind of collaboration did not sufficiently understand the science of CHI research to recognize the need for the distinction. While there is now an emerging view that models and studies are ethically different, I argue that it is important to go beyond existing work to more clearly delineate how the application of an ethical framework differs when developing a new model versus using conducting a CHI study.

WHO Guidance

The WHO has released three guidance documents on the ethics of CHI research. The first WHO guidance document on CHI research ethics was published in May 2020 and provided key criteria for CHI studies with SARS-CoV-2 (WHO Working Group, 2020). The second was a more general document to address the full range of CHI research that had been in progress prior to the pandemic (World Health Organization [WHO], 2021). In early 2024, the WHO released a third guidance document that drew lessons learned from the experience of CHI research conducted during the COVID-19 pandemic, with the goal of later developing criteria for the use of CHI research during future pandemics (WHO, 2024). Although all three documents use slightly different criteria, the final guidance document attempted to harmonize ethical considerations across these documents and develop a more parsimonious list of ethical criteria (Table 4.1). Nothing was eliminated, but some criteria that previously stood alone were combined, such as consultation, coordination, and public engagement.

Some differences between the guidance documents are likely attributable to the fact that they have different goals. The first key criteria document was rapidly developed during the early days of the COVID-19 pandemic to address the use of CHI research on an emerging infectious disease, while the most recent is intended to build on that document and include lessons learned from the pandemic. The document produced in the interim provides more general guidance meant to apply across pathogens and not just in emergencies. Accordingly, some considerations provided in the general guidance for CHI research that are typically addressed by standard review processes and may not be distinct for CHI research were left out of the pandemic-focused documents (e.g., payment, privacy, and confidentiality).

Yet, in all of these documents, the ethically relevant differences between developing a new CHI model versus conducting a CHI study with an established model have not been made explicit. For example, the 2024 guidance document notes that a "CHI study must have especially compelling scientific justification during public health emergencies." It is not clear whether this is meant to hold for the creation of a new model during a public health emergency or any CHI research designed to address the public health emergency. For instance, the UK's common cold unit had investigated coronaviruses for many years and developed models with coronaviruses that were related to SARS-CoV-2, such as coronavirus 229E (Tyrrell, 1992). Presumably, a CHI study with an existing model that used a cold-inducing coronavirus strain and had an established record of safety could have been conducted during the COVID-19 pandemic without such scrutiny (Callow et al., 1990).

The WHO guidance also provides procedural criteria for CHI research that would also benefit from greater recognition of the difference between models and studies. The two procedural criteria are (1) expert review and (2) coordination, consultation, and public engagement. For example, one point of contention in the literature has been whether CHI research should undergo standard review processes or whether additional review by a specially constituted committee with relevant expertise is needed. The WHO document indicates that special review is needed for CHI research during an emergency but that, if the

Table 4.1 WHO criteria for controlled human infection (CHI) research across guidance documents with proposed consolidation of criteria

	Key criteria for COVID (2020)	Key criteria for future pandemics (2024)	General guidance for CHI research (2022)	Proposed consolidated criteria
1	Scientific justification	Scientific justification	Justification	Sufficient social value
2	Assessment of risks and potential benefits	Assessment of risks and potential benefits	Risks, burdens, and benefits Research design	Reasonable risk/benefit profile
3	Consultation and engagement	Coordination, consultation, and engagement		Engagement of relevant parties
4	Coordination		Data management and sharing	
5	Site selection	Site selection	Site selection	Suitable site selection
6	Participant selection	Participant selection	Participant selection	Fair participant selection
7	Expert review	Expert review	Review and oversight	Expert review
8	Informed consent	Informed consent	Consent and notification	Robust informed consent
9			Privacy and confidentiality	[addressed in risk]
10			Reimbursement, compensation, & incentives	Proportionate payment

initial studies do not produce "unexpected harms or public concerns specific to the research," subsequent CHI research with the pathogen could be reviewed under standard approaches. This approach may be both under- and overinclusive. Harms that are expected but more severe than anticipated might merit a slower and more careful process.

For a pathogen that evolves rapidly, such as SARS-CoV-2, there may be a need to develop multiple novel CHI models with different strains, each of which might require extra scrutiny. Even the first study with a CHI model to test vaccines or treatments that are themselves not well understood might benefit from special review.

Additionally, public engagement might have different requirements for models and studies. Public concerns can span a large range of responses, from fringe concerns to fears among large numbers of people that decrease their trust in CHI research, research in general, or vaccines. Consultation and engagement were very important before creating a new CHI model with SARS-CoV-2, both because of the many complex ethical issues it raised and also because of the heated debate over whether developing the model could affect public trust in research. Once the initial model had been developed, however, it is not clear whether the same level of consultation and engagement was required for the use of that model in CHI studies in the United Kingdom, particularly because initial studies had not suggested there was substantial public concern about CHI research in that setting.

A more principled way to determine when special protections or extra effort are needed is to distinguish between the development of a new CHI model and the use of a model that has been proved safe and reliable in CHI studies. If, for instance, researchers keep creating new models with different strains of the pathogen or related pathogens, additional protections might continue to be necessary. But once the models are demonstrated to be safe, using them to test vaccines or treatments might be much less ethically complicated. As discussed further below, distinguishing models from studies is important because it clarifies that the creation of new models requires special attention to the greater ethical complexity, which may require an additional layer of review beyond the standard approach.

Eight Ethical Criteria for Conducting Controlled Human Infection Research

After reviewing existing guidance and ethical literature, eight ethical criteria emerge that can capture the concerns raised by CHI research.

Six of these criteria are substantive—focused on what is being done in the research—and two are procedural—focused on what processes the research should go through before being conducted (Table 4. 2). I will go through each criterion in turn, with special attention to the distinction between CHI models and CHI studies with respect to social value, risk, and independent review. For the other criteria, the differences between CHI models and CHI studies are not as substantial, but I delineate key differences in each subsection as appropriate.

Sufficient Social Value

The first step in justifying a challenge model or study requires measuring the potential value that CHI research offers for society (or "social value") to ensure it has sufficient value to proceed. Biomedical research has social value when it uses sound methods to address important questions related to health (Council for International Organizations of Medical Sciences, 2016). Social value is a function of the importance of the potential benefit, the likelihood that it will be realized, and how that benefit is distributed (Rid & Roestenberg, 2020). All research should have social value to be ethically justifiable, and research that poses risks to participants and third parties requires sufficient social value to justify those risks (Wendler & Rid, 2017). Social value can be difficult to measure for CHI research, however, as it generally functions as a complement to other types of research (Rid & Roestenberg, 2020).

Determining whether CHI research has sufficient social value also requires comparing the expected value to the value of alternative approaches to learning similar information, including other research in humans and animals. While CHI research has many unique attributes and can often produce rich and precise data about things like the timing of infection, symptoms, and infectiousness, such precision may not always be worth the burdens and risks, depending on whether similar knowledge can be gained with a different approach.

One key alternative to CHI research is the use of challenge studies with animals, including but not limited to nonhuman primates (Barnhill et al., 2016; DeGrazia & Miller, 2021). A recent article from

Table 4.2 Ethical criteria for controlled human infection (CHI) research distinguishing models from studies

Type of criteria	Consolidated criteria	Application to CHIMs	Application to CHIS
Substantive	1. Sufficient social value	More rigorous assessment of social value is needed to account for additional uncertainty in CHI models & downstream uses.	Social value is clearer but more limited, important to evaluate social value of intervention being tested in CHI studies along with other scientific questions.
	2. Reasonable risk–benefit profile	Risks may be unusually uncertain, so robust justification is needed for parameters affecting risk, e.g., choice of strain, initial dose, dose escalation, ways to minimize third party risks, plans for compensation for research-related injury.	Risk assessment can focus on safety data from CHI model and any proposed deviations from model that might modify risks/benefits (e.g., less monitoring or confinement), along with risk/benefit from any interventions being tested.
	3. Suitable site selection	Clear justification is needed for initial choice of site. Models should generally not be created in sites with limited CHI experience, lack of capacity to manage disease under study according to an ethically acceptable standard of care.	If CHI study is being done in same site as model, no new questions may arise. If done in a different site, important to evaluate site-level factors.
	4. Fair participant selection	The choice of participants should minimize risk/burden while also considering relevant population for future intervention.	If CHI study is being done in same population as model, no new questions are likely to arise. If in a different population, need to consider risks/burdens & benefits.

Table 4.2 Continued

Type of criteria	Consolidated criteria	Application to CHIMs	Application to CHIS
	5. Robust informed consent	The process should use robust, evidence-based approach to ensure understanding of greater uncertainty of value and risk, third party risks, and restrictions on participant liberty.	Standard approaches to informed consent may suffice with some enhancement (e.g., tests of understanding).
	6. Proportionate payment	There is no major distinction between models and studies; standard payment approaches should be used.	See previous column.
Procedural	7. Engagement of relevant parties	It is important to engage communities prior to creation of model to address risks to participants, potential threats to public trust & third-party risks. Embedded ethics/ social science research may be beneficial.	Community input and dialogue is generally helpful, but additional engagement may be needed if the study is being done in new sites/populations.
	8. Expert review	The creation of new models typically requires additional layer of review, and should involve reviewers with expertise in CHI research and/or the pathogen being studied.	Standard REC/ IRB review should suffice; consultation with experts on CHI research or the pathogen may still be beneficial.

David DeGrazia and Frank Miller helpfully draws on a new framework for animal research ethics to provide a more rigorous analysis of the ethical issues that also represents an attempt at achieving as much agreement as possible among people on opposite sides of the debate over animal research, biomedical researchers, and animal protection advocates. While a full discussion of the ethics of animal challenge studies goes beyond the scope of this book, it is worth noting that both of these articles ultimately concluded that there could be conditions where CHI research with humans would not be ethically acceptable but infection challenge research with nonhuman primates might be if it is to save the lives of humans (DeGrazia & Miller, 2021). A potential argument to the contrary is that non-human animals cannot give their consent to authorize their participation in research, suggesting that it would be more ethically permissible to conduct CHI research than infection challenge research with animals. Another critical question is whether it is possible to extrapolate from the animal model of a particular disease to humans, and, to the extent that particular animals have a very different disease course than humans, animal infection challenge models may not be suitable alternatives to CHI research. Miller and DeGrazia acknowledge the growing concern over the use of some animal models that have limited, if any, translation to human disease (van der Worp et al., 2010) and argue that it is important to ensure that an animal model is a scientifically valid alternative to research with humans, in addition to understanding the level of social value it can generate, in order to justify its conduct.

So far, this discussion has not required distinguishing CHI models from CHI studies, but the rest of this section will clarify how social value considerations apply differently to CHI models versus CHI studies.

Social Value for CHI Models

The social value of CHI models comes from two main sources. First, the primary endpoint of a CHI model is to develop a reproducible and safe way of infecting most of the people exposed to the strain. Participants are followed very closely between exposure and infection. For these reasons, CHI models are very useful for yielding scientific insights about the course of disease. For example, CHI models are a good way to study the early course of disease, when most people are unaware that they are sick and do not typically present to care. CHI models can help identify or refine correlates of protection, which are biological markers that can demonstrate when someone has protection from becoming infected, such as antibody levels. CHI models can also include other secondary endpoints, such as testing how a virus spreads within a room or the effectiveness of different tests for infection. Second, once a CHI model has been created, it can be used to test vaccines or therapeutic interventions in a controlled, relatively fast, and reliable way. The downstream benefits of developing a new CHI model can therefore be substantial but are also highly uncertain and dependent on many factors, including the epidemiology of a disease when the CHI model is ready for use.

The clearest example of high social value from developing a CHI model occurs when there are no good alternatives to the CHI model for answering the scientific question at hand. For example, in rare cases, the downstream benefits of CHI studies with an established CHI model can be useful as the primary way interventions are tested if it is not feasible to test the intervention in field trials—as has been the case for Zika virus, where outbreaks became too unpredictable and sporadic to support field trials (Vannice et al., 2019). Because CHI models and CHIs typically use artificial approaches to infecting small numbers of participants who are often very homogenous, they are rarely sufficient to test whether something will work in the real world with diverse groups of people. Rather, in most cases, CHI studies testing interventions are used as a complement to other research. For example, CHI studies with malaria have been used to prioritize among different treatments and vaccine candidates that then go on to be tested in the field (Roestenberg et al., 2018).

On the other hand, evaluating CHI models when there are alternatives to learning similar, if not the same, information can be more challenging. This is because review committees must assess the short-term value of learning about the early stages of disease along with the longer-term, more attenuated value that might (or might not) manifest in several different ways. One example is the creation of a CHI model for HCV. HCV is well understood and can be treated successfully with highly effective direct-acting antivirals (Geddawy et al.,

2017). Given low access to diagnostics and treatment and the fact that there is a risk of reinfection after successful treatment, it is thought that an HCV vaccine will be important to eradicate the virus (Rid et al., 2023). There are several candidates in development, and the ability to test them in an HCV CHI model might help to speed up vaccine testing. The value of a CHI model for HCV might be one of the keys that leads toward eradication of the virus at some point in the future. On the other hand, the fact that there are available effective treatments suggest that the value of conducting an HCV CHI model might also be lower than that for creating a CHI model for other diseases, particularly if other ways to test vaccines might exist but take longer than the use of a CHI model.

Social Value of CHI Studies with an Established Model

CHI studies have more direct social value than CHI models but make more focused, less pluripotent contributions to society than CHI models. The social value of a particular CHI study depends on the intervention being tested in the study along with any other scientific questions the study is addressing. This can be substantial, as in the case of a Zika CHI study that is the only way to test a Zika vaccine, but it is also inherently less valuable than the creation of the initial CHI model.

While an initial assessment of social value is important to ensure a study should be conducted in the first place, the next consideration in evaluating the ethics of CHI models and CHI studies is the risk level, to ensure that the risk is outweighed by the potential social value.

Reasonable Risk–Benefit Profile

In any research study, including CHI research, risks to participants and third parties should be identified, minimized, and justified before the study is deemed acceptable. This includes longer-term risks of harm, and compensation for research-related injury is important to remove barriers to the treatment and care needed to minimize risks. The uncertainty surrounding risks of harm are qualitatively different in creating a new CHI model as opposed to conducting CHI studies;

this uncertainty diminishes over time as greater experience with a model accrues.

Importantly, while some have contended that a rescue therapy is necessary for CHI research to be ethically acceptable (Weijer, 2024), the presence or absence of a rescue treatment is merely one part of the analysis of risk and should not be required. Some diseases are likely to resolve on their own, without lasting effects, so long as people receive medical attention and have access to supportive care, such as intravenous fluids. Not all CHI models are created equal in this regard. While CHI studies with malaria infect participants with a drug-susceptible strain of malaria and then treat them, CHI models developed for cholera, Dengue, and influenza lack specific treatments for the disease. Cholera is an illness that is likely to completely resolve with adequate supportive care, and conducting CHI studies with cholera generally raises limited ethical concerns. For Dengue and influenza, it is less certain that all participants can be restored to their initial state of health, and these were some of the riskiest examples of CHI research prior to the creation of the model for SARS-CoV-2 during the COVID-19 pandemic.

Additionally, participant selection is an important way to minimize risk. For many pathogens, people who are young and otherwise healthy are unlikely to have serious complications. There may be some risk factors, genetic or otherwise, that predispose healthy people to serious reactions, but if those are widely known, then the risk level of CHI research can be very low even without a rescue treatment. Another issue is that it is not clear what "rescue" is meant to refer to. The term "rescue" implies that a participant is in grave danger and is pulled back from the abyss by the treatment. However, some treatments may only work well when administered early in the course of disease to reduce the severity of symptoms and reduce the risk of death substantially, such as monoclonal antibodies in the COVID pandemic. The use of treatments that reduce risk, combined with careful participant selection, may be sufficient to render the risk of CHI research minimal. Thus, the risk–benefit ratio is the critical component for evaluation, not the presence or absence of a rescue therapy.

Reasonable Risk–Benefit Profile in CHI Models

Just as creating a new CHI model requires identifying a method for infection that is safe enough for use, there are also many components of the process that are focused on safety and minimizing risk. To identify and minimize risk, researchers need to select a facility with enough security to prevent transmission of the pathogen to the environment, select a strain that is useful for testing future interventions but not likely to cause severe harms, develop protections for research personnel to ensure that they are not infected, determine whether and how long participants should be confined to prevent infection of others and allow for close monitoring of symptoms, and decide what types of care and/or treatment the research participants will receive. Strains typically must undergo a process of purification, which could follow Good Manufacturing Practice processes or some other process to verify that participants are receiving the pathogen in question and not anything else that could cause harm. This is important to minimize the risk that participants are being infected with pathogens other than the one the researchers intend to use.

Additionally, the selection of the initial dose is also important for the level of risk and uncertainty. A dose that is too high could lead to symptoms on the more severe end of the spectrum, even with people who are normally at low risk. While the question of which dose to use to begin is challenging, this uncertainty is somewhat mitigated by taking a careful approach to titrating the dose and starting with a very low dose that is not likely to make people very sick, potentially even doses that are so low as to be at homeopathic levels. As will be discussed in Chapter 5, how much is known about the pathogen can also add to the uncertainty. The initial dose that was used in the SARS-CoV-2 CHI model was 1/10 of the dose recommended by the WHO's technical working group (Levine et al., 2020), but it was sufficient to infect most of the participants and cause one participant to have extended loss of smell and taste (Killingley et al., 2022). It is unclear what would have happened if the researchers had started with the dose that the WHO's experts had recommended.

In general, if the pathogen is something that has been infecting people for decades or centuries, as with an HCV CHI model, there is more certainty about the potential side effects and possible complications after infection based on robust epidemiologic data. As long as a strain was selected that was likely to respond to treatment and participants were treated before long-term consequences could emerge, an HCV CHI model poses less risk and uncertainty than other CHI models (Rid et al., 2023). For emerging infectious diseases like SARS-CoV-2 in 2020, however, the uncertainty surrounding the dose was compounded by limited knowledge about who was at risk and what the risks might have been. Researchers can also plan to enroll people who are likely at low risk of serious complications from the pathogen; again, this is easier to do with diseases that are well understood.

While minimizing risk is critical, there can be tradeoffs between the risk level and the scientific knowledge that will result. There may be some cases where it is justifiable not to minimize risk as far as possible if the risk is reasonable and the importance of the knowledge to be gained is significant. For instance, as assays for detecting malaria become more sensitive, it was possible to begin treating participants in CHI studies with malaria very early in the disease course, which would minimize their risks of experiencing symptoms of malaria. However, very early treatment would make it harder to detect the effects of interventions, and participants could still be cured if they were treated slightly later in their course, once they began having symptoms, but before any lasting impact is likely. Thus, it may be acceptable to delay treatment slightly despite the ability to minimize participant burden by treating them sooner, particularly if the risks are not excessive and can be justified by the increased value.

In addition to identifying, minimizing, and evaluating the risks to participants, risks to third parties not enrolled in the research must also be considered, which will depend on how the pathogen spreads (Shah et al., 2018). Third parties include research personnel and staff, as well as others unconnected to the study who could be infected by the participants. The use of personal protective equipment and careful research procedures can minimize the risks of infecting research staff. In some cases, if the pathogen has the potential to circulate on its own outside of the study, there is a risk of creating local outbreaks as well.

To minimize the risks to third parties in the community, researchers conducting controlled human malaria infection studies sometimes inject the virus rather than relying on mosquitoes to spread it or use facilities that are designed to prevent mosquitos from escaping. Participants are also carefully monitored and treated by a certain point to ensure that they do not spread the disease to others. Researchers may need to ask participants to be confined or to limit contact with people who might be at higher risk to ensure they do not infect third parties outside of the study, although this can add burden to the study for participants (Fernandez Lynch, 2020).

Another potential group harm is that, if a negative outcome occurred in CHI research, there is potential damage to public trust in CHI research in general or other types of research. For example, if a participant were to become severely injured or die in a study involving CHI research that was used to test a vaccine, this could feed into distrust in vaccines. As noted in Chapter 2, the risk of public distrust in research could be even more important if there is a heightened "yuck reaction," which depends, of course, on the model. As noted in Chapter 3, the fact that CHI researchers deliberately infect participants suggests that they have greater moral responsibility if serious harm comes to a participant than do researchers using different methods where infection may be foreseen but is not intended.

When there is a high degree of uncertainty about risk that includes the potential for high risk, either to participants or third parties, CHI models rarely if ever offer a prospect of direct benefit to offset the risks because their goal is simply to infect people with pathogens. One exception to this general rule that will be discussed further in Chapter 6 is CHI research inoculating people with probiotic bacteria that can help protect against infection with other bacteria that cause disease (Deasy et al., 2015). For most CHI research, then, the risks should be weighed against potential benefits to society, as compared with the alternative approaches to learning similar information. This is often done implicitly and may seem difficult to do in a nonarbitrary way. However, some authors have demonstrated how a more systematic approach can be used, particularly when the risks and benefits are highly uncertain (Kuiper et al., 2021; Rid & Roestenberg, 2020; Yu et al., 2020).

Reasonable Risk–Benefit Profile for CHI Studies

For CHI studies, the risks will typically be less uncertain than for CHI models, as they will have been characterized in the CHI model. Depending on the amount of prior experience with the model, the uncertainty could range considerably. Additionally, any choices made in a study to deviate from the model would have to be examined and justified, particularly if these changes could increase the risk. For example, changes that might occur in a study could include less intensive monitoring of participants, which might lead to delay in catching serious complications.

Unlike in the development of a CHI model, the interventions that are being tested in CHI studies will also change the risk–benefit profile. Vaccines and other interventions also pose risks that must be evaluated and may not be fully understood at the time they are tested in CHI studies. For example, the risk of vaccine-enhanced disease was theorized to be a potential risk of SARS-CoV-2 vaccines but one that did not ultimately materialize. Additionally, CHI studies differ from models because they could offer a prospect of direct benefit to participants that should be weighed against the risk. If vaccines being tested in CHI studies have prior efficacy data that suggest participants may receive protection against disease, this could count as a potential benefit from study participation.

Ultimately, CHI studies may have less social value and risk than the creation of a model, but whatever value and risk they do have would typically be more certain. In this way, a CHI study with an established model that has accumulated data demonstrating its safe use might not be able to justify as much net risk to participants as a CHI model, but might have less net risk to begin with and thereby could be easier to evaluate and justify.

Suitable Site Selection

Deciding where to conduct research has not typically been considered a benchmark of ethical research (Emanuel et al., 2000). For the creation of a new CHI model, however, it is critically important to consider where it is being conducted (Shah, Miller & Darton et al., 2020).

A range of factors should be considered in making this determination, such as (1) how much experience the site has with conducting CHI models in general and with CHI models that use the particular type of pathogen; (2) whether there is a robust healthcare system to ensure participants can receive treatment for any longer-term effects of being infected with the pathogen, (3) whether the public health infrastructure can prevent transmission of pathogens or create additional protections if participants withdraw from the study early while infectious (Fernandez Lynch, 2020), (4) how sensitized the community has been to the concept of research in general and CHI research in particular, (5) whether there is experience at the site in treating the particular pathogen that participants will be infected with, (6) the level of risk of burdening an overburdened healthcare system if CHI research participants become very sick, and (7) the existence of a solid research ethics oversight system that can provide rigorous review of the protocol. These factors may not be exhaustive but are critical to manage the ethical complexity involved in creating a new CHI model.

For CHI studies, it might be less important for all these factors to be in place, or it might be clearer which factors are important based on what was learned from the CHI model. For example, CHI studies with established models that do not carry significant risks of long-term harm may be easier to justify and may be a reasonable way for sites to build capacity that could ultimately enable them to develop new CHI models, even if those sites lack a mechanism for addressing long-term harms experienced by research participants, like universal health care.

Fair Participant Selection

Traditionally, fair participant selection was understood to be about choosing who to invite into research based on scientific reasons and not giving special access to research benefits for those who are privileged or taking advantage of vulnerable people by exposing them to excess risk. More recently, Doug MacKay and Kate Saylor have argued that there are actually four components (or "faces") of fair participant selection that can be helpful to consider separately; specifically, (1) fair inclusion, (2) fair burden sharing, (3) fair opportunity, and (4) fair distribution of third-party risks. In CHI research, it is most important to think about fair burden sharing and fair distribution of risks to participants and third parties (MacKay et al., 2020). CHI research typically enrolls small numbers of people who are typically young and healthy under tightly controlled conditions, making it difficult for this research to reflect a diverse population. Inclusion of representative groups does not generally apply to CHI research for this reason. As noted above, CHI research also does not typically offer a prospect of direct benefit because exposure to or infection by a pathogen is usually not beneficial, making it less important to be concerned about fair opportunity to receive the benefits of research and more important to consider the distribution of burdens.

Fair participant selection plays out somewhat differently in CHI models compared to CHI studies. When developing a new CHI model, minimizing the risks and burdens to participants and third parties is critical. This requires careful attention to the choice of participants who are likely to be at lower risk from infection and who are also less likely to infect third parties. The choice of population for a CHI model will provide guidance in future CHI studies. If a CHI study uses an existing model with a population that is very different from the original population enrolled, this may introduce greater uncertainty and a need for more stringent review. For example, use of a CHI model with malaria in people living with HIV was important prior to the rollout of a malaria vaccine (Jongo et al., 2024) but increased the risks of the study and uncertainty about outcomes from the use of an existing model, and therefore it required clear justification and analysis of the ethical issues involved.

One emerging issue about fair selection of participants that has not been discussed much if at all in the literature is that some countries have not conducted CHI models or CHI studies but still reap the benefit when other countries do so. In time, this may lead to a free rider problem where everyone benefits from the scientific knowledge produced, but only some countries and people contribute to the development of that knowledge. This type of concern extends beyond CHI research but may be especially salient in this context, for example, if there is an intuitive negative reaction to CHI research in certain countries that leads to reluctance to create a regulatory pathway to permit such research, and those countries still benefit from the data learned from CHI research conducted in other countries.[1]

Robust Informed Consent

Even among those who question whether CHI research warrants special ethical attention, there is widespread agreement on the importance of informed consent to ensure CHI research is ethical (Steel, 2020). Informed consent requires ensuring that participants have the capacity to understand the research, disclosing relevant information to them that a reasonable person would want to know, ensuring they understand this information, and obtaining their authorization to proceed with the research.

As will be discussed at greater length in Chapter 6, ethicists have largely argued that only adults who have the capacity to make autonomous decisions should be enrolled in CHI research (Bambery et al., 2015; Miller & Grady, 2001). Some have questioned whether there should be a categorical exclusion of children from CHI research and suggested additional safeguards that could make it ethically acceptable to conduct such research (Murphy et al., 2020). Additionally, CHI research has been conducted with inclusion/exclusion criteria that prevent people from participating if they have low literacy levels or are not highly educated, assuming that they would therefore lack capacity to understand the research. Elsewhere, I have argued with others that a lack of education is not necessarily a barrier to understanding and that exclusion of participants based on assumptions about their inability to understand is unjustified. Rather, researchers should make efforts to improve consent processes and test understanding to ensure all participants know what they are getting into when they enroll in CHI research (Vaswani et al., 2020).

There are certain key features of the research that participants should understand before enrolling in CHI research, namely: (1) that they will deliberately be exposed to infectious agents, (2) why the

---

[1] I thank Kenji Matsui for this point.

research is being done and what the potential social value is, (3) the risks and burdens, and (4) any restrictions on their liberty necessary to protect them and third parties (including whether there will be a period of confinement) (Vaswani et al., 2020). Given the degree of commitment required by participants in CHI research, robust approaches to informed consent are critical. Despite many studies testing innovations to the consent process, the two approaches that result in the greatest increases in understanding are allowing individuals more time to go through consent processes in discussion with others and testing people and providing them with feedback for any answers they do not get right the first time (Flory & Emanuel, 2004). Future work on informed consent will likely continue to identify methods for improving understanding and appreciation of research among participants.

Although there is copious literature on informed consent, there has been little attention to the difference between informed consent in CHI models versus CHI studies. In the development of new CHI models, the use of the best evidence in developing a robust informed consent process is arguably even more critical in CHI model development as opposed to the use of established models in CHI study. It is also critical that participants understand the limitations of CHI models and that, if they are enrolled in research to develop a model, they will not be contributing directly to testing interventions or receiving vaccines. Data from those who signed on to a registry to participate in CHI research to address COVID-19 suggest that there can be substantial confusion among participants between a model and a study (Marsh et al., 2022). Furthermore, tests of understanding used in CHI models might benefit from strict standards to ensure that anyone who participates is able to understand the information at a high level.

Proportionate Payment

There has been a fair amount of attention to the ethics of payment in CHI research (Anomaly & Savulescu, 2019; Grimwade et al., 2020; Lynch et al., 2021). Some have argued for a model that could involve substantial amounts of payment for participants in CHI research, suggesting that "any amount" that is needed to recruit and retain participants would be ethical given the anticipation of high risk and social value (Anomaly & Savulescu, 2019). Others have argued that payment for CHI research can be high but should be proportionate to the risk of harm (Anomaly & Savulescu, 2019; Grimwade et al., 2020). On the other hand, a comprehensive overview of payment in the context of CHI research led by Holly Lynch concluded that CHI research is not unique with respect to payment and that claims of the higher potential for risk and social value are not fully borne out (2021). This leads Lynch and colleagues to conclude that a standard framework for ethical payment in research can equally be applied to CHI research, although the application of the framework reveals some important considerations for CHI research.

Lynch and colleagues separate payment into three categories: reimbursement for actual and reasonable expenses, compensation, and incentives. They argue that reimbursement raises no ethical concerns because such payments are revenue-neutral and do not benefit participants; reimbursement should therefore be provided as a matter of course to participants. After all, if participants are not reimbursed for their expenses, they would effectively be subsidizing the research. Compensation for time, burden, and inconvenience should also be offered to participants as a matter of fairness but should be examined because it can raise the potential for exploitation if it is not sufficient and undue inducement if it is excessive. Finally, incentives go beyond reimbursing participants or compensating them for their time, and therefore go beyond what fairness requires. Incentives are more controversial, in part because of misconceptions about the coercive potential of payments (Wertheimer & Miller, 2008) that will be discussed further below, but they are important at times to increase the number and pool of people who will consider participating in research.

Views about payment for research participation, and participation in CHI research in particular, typically fall on a spectrum. At one end of the spectrum, some people view payment as morally problematic, if sometimes a necessary evil. For example, one CHI study in Colombia did not pay volunteers for their participation at all, based on concerns that payment would attract people who are doing research for the wrong reasons. Although the researchers screened many participants to find enough to participate, they were ultimately able to carry out the study (Herrera et al., 2009). Similarly, as noted in Chapter 6, the initial draft of guidance from the Indian Council of Medical Research on CHI research required that participants be altruistically motivated and planned not to inform participants how much they would be paid until after they agreed to participate. Whether these plans would really ensure altruism is questionable—it seems easy for participants to indicate that they are altruistically motivated even if they are not or if their motives are mixed, which is common for CHI participants. Additionally, how much participants were going to be paid would be unlikely to remain secret once some people knew about it. And if someone enrolled but found out how much they were being paid and thought it was too little, they could always withdraw from the research immediately afterward.

Others who are concerned about payment have a more measured approach to their concerns. While they recognize that it is important for volunteers to be reimbursed for expenses and compensated for their time, some believe it is important that volunteers should not be paid too much, or it would serve as an undue inducement. The worry seems to be that too much money would blind people to the risks involved, compromise their deeply held values and beliefs, or encourage them to withhold information the researchers need to know that might disqualify them from participation. Concerns about undue inducement can be evaluated with empirical evidence to some degree. The first concern—that money blinds people to risks—is not borne out by data. One study suggests that people who are motivated by money spend more time evaluating the risks and understand them better (Cryder et al., 2010). Other studies found that, for some people, high amounts of payment simply would not entice them to participate, particularly when higher payment means higher risk (Halpern et al., 2021; Hoogerwerf et al., 2020). Additionally, making sure that participants demonstrate their understanding through a test/feedback approach to informed consent (Flory & Emanuel, 2004), as is frequently done in CHI research (Vaswani et al., 2020), is one way to address this worry. Perhaps the concern is that people will understand the risks but take on more risk than they should based on some notion of the upper limit of risk. Notably, this is a type of hard paternalism that should be owned up to and addressed by delineating what that upper limit of risk should be. It also would presumably be addressed by Institutional Review Boards (IRBs) that review the research to make sure it is ethically sound. In research with groups such as pregnant people and children, existing regulations put into place risk limits that would presumably prevent research with excessive risks from being approved in the first place (Murphy et al., 2020).

The second concern about people compromising their values and beliefs is harder to evaluate empirically. We tried to evaluate this concern in a small qualitative study of participants in a malaria CHI. Most participants indicated that study participation did not conflict with their values or beliefs. However, one participant did describe a similar concern as follows: "The biggest qualm that I had was a personal thing in that I don't take medicine. I don't do any drugs or alcohol. . . . So the idea of sacrificing that habit for one time . . . I kind of had to think" (Kraft et al., 2019). The study would require being infected with malaria (which did not conflict with his habit) and then being treated with malarone (which did come into conflict with his general views). When pressed on this, however, he said it is just a "practice" that he generally adheres to, and it felt fine to make an exception in this case, so it did not indicate he had compromised his deepest values by participating in CHI research. It is hard to find examples of this concern and to know whether it is appropriate for an observer to raise an objection because of the subjective nature of values and beliefs. People weigh even deeply held values and beliefs against other considerations all the time, and even religious beliefs often come with exceptions. A Hindu who does not eat beef might still take a life-saving medication derived from bovine products without moral qualms. So while the notion of an "indecent proposal" is one that has a fair amount of cultural valence, it seems difficult to know from the outside whether someone is compromising a belief that they hold sacred in a way that is harmful to them or whether they are simply making a tradeoff that makes sense given the value they place on this belief and their other competing values and interests.

Finally, at the other end of the spectrum, people think that undue inducement is "nonsense on stilts" and that ethicists and review committees should not worry about payment for research participation. Zeke Emanuel argues that if research has gone through a rigorous review process and has been deemed acceptable by a review board, paying participants a large amount of money to join that study won't transform it into something that is unethical (2005). Others go even farther and argue that people should be paid as much as is needed to offset the risk of research (Grimwade et al., 2020). Paying large amounts of money, in their view, is a good thing that ensures enrollment in risky research that might have great value. Lynch and colleagues (2021) argue to the contrary that there may be some reasonable concerns about payment that are not fully allayed by IRB review. Furthermore, paying people for risk upfront requires paying everyone the same amount discounted based on the probability of harm. This means that some people who will not be injured will receive compensation merely for having taken on the risk, and others who are injured will not be fully compensated for the harm they experience. They argue that rather than paying people for risk up front, it is better to ensure there is no-fault compensation for harm for those who experience it. Thus, focusing on compensation after injury rather than risk up front is preferable to address the ethical concern that a person who harms another has a duty to attempt to make the victim whole again (Pike, 2012).

Another worry about payment is that paying high amounts for research participation could lead to an "arms race" of sorts, where some studies struggle to enroll because others pay such large amounts.[2] Anecdotally, I have heard from CHI researchers that this issue sometimes hampers CHI research because Phase I studies run by pharmaceutical companies sometimes pay participants more and ask less of them. The idea that allowing the market to drive what participants are paid could skew enrollment into valuable research is a valid concern. Institutions and ethics review committees could address this worry by having local standards for payment that are applied uniformly and are fairly across studies.

There is another concern specific to CHI research that has received limited attention in the literature to date. While there is no

---

[2] I thank an anonymous reviewer for this point.

clear evidence that payment compromises understanding of the risks involved, there is reason to worry that people might withhold information that could make them ineligible if they are highly motivated to participate. And money is not the only motivation—participants in CHI studies, like participants in other types of research, often mention altruism or a mix of motivations. Some people even do it out of curiosity or a desire for new experiences (Kraft et al., 2019). The challenge is how to figure out whether people who are highly motivated to participate are willing to cross ethical lines for money. In our small study of volunteers in a controlled human malaria infection study, we struggled with the right way to ask people if they were willing to lie for money. We ultimately asked participants if they thought other people would deceive researchers for the money, and most of them thought others might withhold information about drug or alcohol use to ensure they were able to participate. They also noted that participants might not want to share information about stigmatizing or illegal behavior with researchers and that would be another reason that they would not admit to behavior that could disqualify them from participating (Kraft et al., 2019).

Next, we asked if they had withheld any information, not expecting that anyone would admit to it. However, we had designed the study to involve interviews over the phone hoping that people would be more likely to share information that cast them in a negative light in this way. Some people said that they were truthful about things that they were worried would disqualify them from participating and were relieved when they were still able to participate. However, one participant did admit to not following the rules. One of the requirements for being in the study was to use condoms to prevent pregnancy. This participant said that his long-term partner was on birth control pills, and they were not using condoms during the study. He acknowledged that there was a risk of pregnancy and said that they accepted that risk and would not blame the researchers if something were to happen (Kraft et al., 2019).

Another controlled human malaria infection study that was conducted in Kenya had similar findings. In this study, participants were paid for each day they remained in confinement. Once they developed symptoms of malaria, however, they would be treated and sent home. The longer they could go without reporting symptoms, the more money they would receive. The authors noted that while some participants felt it was important to be honest so they could be treated as soon as possible, this was not the case for everyone. Within one cohort, there was almost a competition to "make it to the end" and not report symptoms as long as possible, presumably to make as much money as possible (Chi et al., 2022).

Instead of focusing on restricting payment amounts, there are other, potentially more effective ways researchers can design studies to try to limit deception from participants. First, researchers could appeal to participants not to withhold information and make it clear why it matters, both scientifically and regarding public perception of the research, that people who participate are able to recover and not become any sicker than is necessary. This requires honesty about not meeting exclusion criteria that could make people more vulnerable than the average and about when someone is having symptoms that require treatment. Another approach would be to hide what excludes people from the study, making it harder for people to game the system. In other words, researchers could make it harder for participants to figure out what to lie about. Relatedly, exclusion or treatment criteria could be focused on more objective measures, like lab values and tests to measure if someone is either ineligible or infected, rather than relying on participants to tell researchers that information. For information about past medical conditions, researchers could obtain access to people's medical records and find that information out directly.

But taking money out of the equation entirely, as the Colombian researchers once did, seems not only unnecessary but also ethically problematic, with the potential for unintended consequences. Failing to pay people for participation would in effect be asking them to subsidize the research. Participants in research who cannot do their day jobs need some compensation. Compensating people for the time and burdens they take on is a way of showing respect for their time and contributions. Making sure that they receive care if they become sick is not only important as a matter of respect, but also to minimize the risk that their illness will get worse and lead to long-lasting consequences. Yet this points to another problem with CHI research: some effects of illness can take a very long time to manifest, and research funding is typically bounded in time. Research grants typically last no more than 5 years. While some researcher might purchase insurance to compensate injured or sick participants, even that will come with time limits. What can researchers do to compensate participants who experience consequences from their study participation many years down the line?

Sydney Halpern has noted that participants in hepatitis challenge studies in the 1950s could have experienced effects of infection years later, including liver damage, liver cancer, or even death (2021). Participants with liver cancer could hardly go back to the research team and ask for compensation at that moment. And any pathogen that is not well-understood could lead to similar issues that researchers and participants may not even know to anticipate. The long-term effects of SARS-CoV-2 infection are not fully known. The other problem is that, with the passage of many years, other influences on the course of a person's health will inevitably emerge. People who were infected with SARS-CoV-2 in the UK CHI model might have been infected again after the study. If they developed long COVID at some point, the study was only one potential contributor to that.

Notably, however, the United Kingdom has one key advantage over many other countries in that it has a National Health Service. Any participants who experience long-term complications have a place to go for care and are not expected to bear the burden of illness entirely on their own. In the United States and many other countries, the lack of a national healthcare system makes it much more challenging to address long-term consequences of infection, making it important to purchase insurance to compensate people for harm if it occurs, although this is an imperfect solution. The time-limited nature of insurance connected to a specific study may make it difficult to ensure participants receive care if complications materialize in the longer term.

Engagement of Relevant Parties

Community engagement is widely recognized as important for accomplishing many different goals. While some think engaging communities is intrinsically valuable and worth doing for its own sake, others point to the instrumental reasons that communities should be engaged, several of which apply to CHI research (Shah, Miller & Fernandez Lynch, 2020).

The first step in community engagement is to identify the type of community. Engaging various publics can be important for addressing those who might be at heightened risk of being infected by study participants, to determine the best ways to minimize third-party risks. Engaging with communities could also reveal hidden burdens that should be addressed or inoculate research against rumors that could turn members of the public against these types of studies or research in general (Shah, Miller & Fernandez Lynch, 2020).

Developing a CHI model typically requires more engagement than simply applying an existing model in a CHI study, given the greater uncertainty and ethical complexity. Additionally, in places where prior community engagement about CHI research has not already occurred, more engagement may be needed, particularly if the idea of CHI research is still foreign and likely to trigger a "yuck" reaction, as discussed in Chapter 2.

Members of the public are just one type of community that may be relevant for CHI research. For example, regulators must determine whether results from CHI research could be used to approve the vaccines or treatments that were tested. If regulators are skeptical of this type of research or require field testing, this would be a barrier to translating the research into practice. Advance consultation with regulators could be helpful, particularly during the development of a new CHI model, and can help to ensure that the results will be useful in getting vaccines or treatments approved and available.

Typically, CHI research feeds into other studies in order to lead to product approval, suggesting that other researchers are also key people with whom to engage in advance. The exception that proves the rule is a traveler's cholera vaccine, where the US Food and Drug Administration relied on CHI research only after field trials were too difficult to conduct, and a Zika virus CHI model that the FDA initially expressed skepticism about but ultimately decided was critical for advancing a Zika vaccine when field trials failed because outbreaks would quickly arise and burn out. CHI studies are typically used for prioritizing the best candidates for further testing. Therefore, for most CHI research, it may also be advisable to consult with other researchers who are conducting field trials to see if these results will be valuable to them on the timeline that they are expected. If it will take too long to produce results from a CHI model and the subsequent study with that model for those results to be used in field trials, there may not be much value in developing the model in the first place. Additionally, researchers might want CHI studies to be used to test certain products rather than others, to measure efficacy in a particular way, or to look for certain kinds of safety issues.

Other groups who could be valuable to engage in advance of conducting CHI research could include public health officials who might be able to provide guidance on laws that could interact with the research (such as quarantine requirements) or on how best to implement findings from CHI research about how long diseases incubate or how they are likely to be transmitted.

Finally, the method of engagement can take different forms and should be designed to achieve whatever the goals of engagement happen to be. While the WHO's 2021 guidance document calls out embedded social science research as a form of required engagement, I would argue this is merely one form of engagement that can allow participants' or others' views and experiences to be collected and learned from in a more systematic way. This form of engagement may be especially valuable for new models, but it should not necessarily be required. For example, embedded social science could help to rigorously capture public concerns about the use of a particular type of model or to learn more about participants' experiences and ways to minimize the risks and burdens that they find most challenging to bear.

For CHI studies, community engagement can be important depending on the level of understanding of research in general and of CHI research in the community, the anticipated "yuck" reaction, and the level of risk to third parties, including the need to understand community behavior to mitigate that risk. As a general matter, robust community engagement is more important for CHI models than CHI study with an established model.

Expert Review

Independent review from an IRB or one of its international equivalents is a standard requirement for most research unless it falls into the category of being exempt from regulation because the risk is low and interaction with participants is minimal if not nonexistent. One of the key debates about CHI research is whether standard review is sufficient for this type of research. To answer this question, it is critical to distinguish between two things. First is the difference between developing a new CHI model for the first time and applying a CHI model that has been shown to be safe in a CHI study. Second, there are different types of expert review, including IRB review that includes consultation with experts who are not on the IRB, review by a specialized committee that supplements or supplants IRB review, and ongoing review by a Data Monitoring Committee (DMC) of unblinded data as a study is being conducted.

As argued previously, if a new CHI model is being developed, many parameters of the model will need to be set to ensure it is safe and reproducible. This includes the selection of the site and facility, the precautions being used to prevent third parties from being infected, and the strain of the pathogen that will be used to infect participants. These components should be evaluated by a committee that has the expertise to evaluate safety and scientific validity. IRBs may or may not have the capacity and expertise to evaluate these parameters of a new CHI model. If they do not have the expertise in reviewing CHI models, then one approach would be to consult with experts temporarily for the purpose of evaluating the study, as suggested by Bambery and colleagues (2015). However, for a CHI model that presents many complex and unresolved issues, a specialized committee might be necessary, as was done for the SARS-CoV-2 CHI models (Williams et al., 2022) and a Zika CHI model before that (Shah et al., 2017).

Another important parameter that is set during the development of a new CHI model is the dose of the pathogen and the way that dose is administered or given to participants. Typically, a new CHI model will begin with a lower dose than seems to be necessary to infect most participants, without making them too sick. A DMC is often an important protection to have in place as the dose is slowly escalated because the DMC is comprised of expert clinicians, statisticians, and some-times ethicists who are external to the study and have some objectivity. The DMC can quickly determine if there are concerns about escalating a dose or if it is safe to keep going to get to the level that will infect most of the participants.

For CHI studies that use established models in essentially the way that the CHI model was designed (i.e., without changing the parameters substantially) specialized review would arguably not be necessary, and the standard approach to review might be suffi-cient. IRBs or their international equivalents can use existing ethical frameworks to guide their review, review the data from the existing CHI model, and focus their attention on ways that the CHI study departs from the model, even if it is only that the CHI study involves testing an intervention that changes the risk-benefit ratio of the study.

Conclusion

In recent years, scholars have devoted long-overdue attention to ad-dress the ethics of CHI research. I have argued that use of an ethical framework with eight criteria can help evaluate whether CHI research is ethically acceptable. This framework recognizes the level of uncer-tainty accompanying the creation of a new CHI model, along with the impact of the decisions made at the model stage in all future CHI studies, and therefore requires increased ethical scrutiny for a new CHI model.

There may be other circumstances where additional scrutiny or re-view is helpful for CHI study, as when an existing model is used in a novel way that increases the risk and uncertainty. For example, the ini-tial controlled human malaria infection studies that were conducted in low- and middle-income countries that had no prior experience with this type of research may be a situation requiring extra ethical atten-tion, or when such studies enrolled people living with HIV. In these cases, additional justification and scrutiny similar to that which would accompany the development of a new model may be appropriate. There may also be some cases where a new model requires limited if any additional scrutiny if it involves a pathogen that is very well known and characterized, and the study is designed to take a conservative approach to risk on any parameters that remain uncertain.

Finally, while all criteria are relevant for models and studies, and the specific ways the criteria are distinct for the creation of a new model (or a riskier extension of an existing model) have been elaborated above, there is also another important way that the framework can help ensure the ethics of CHI research. The burden of proof for showing a given criteria has been met is typically higher when justifying a new model than when evaluating the use of an established model in a CHI study that does not add additional risk

Acknowledgments

This chapter in particular benefited greatly from conversations with Annette Rid about existing ethical frameworks and their limitations, in addition to the work I did with her and others to develop an ethical framework that grounds this analysis. Additionally, although this chapter contains my own views on the WHO guidance documents and ICMR document, I contributed to the WHO guidance documents and provided peer review of the ICMR document upon request.

5

CHI Research with Emerging Infectious Diseases

> Q: What was your first reaction to the idea of a COVID-19 infection study?
>
> A: I understood why they're normally unethical (I remember learning about abuses like the Tuskegee Experiment in school). But given the catastrophe we're in, I thought it seemed like an obviously good idea, and the idea that somebody out there is pushing for it actually gave me some hope.
>
> —Interview with a volunteer for 1Day Sooner

In December 2019, some patients in the city of Wuhan, China, experienced symptoms of a respiratory illness that did not respond to standard treatments. By the end of the month, the Chinese office of the World Health Organization (WHO) received reports that there were several patients experiencing pneumonia without a clear cause. On January 5, a Chinese virologist named Yong-Zhen Zhang from Fudan University in Shanghai submitted the genetic sequence for the virus that was infecting patients to Chinese health officials. Two days later, Chinese public health officials identified that a new coronavirus was the cause of this apparent outbreak. The genetic sequence of the virus was published on January 10, 2020, and, by mid-January, several countries reported cases of the novel coronavirus within their borders. On January 23, 2020, the Chinese government instituted a lockdown of Wuhan, a city of 13 million people. Countries began instituting quarantine orders for people who had flown out of Wuhan, China. In February, the WHO officially named the disease "Coronavirus Disease 2019," or "COVID-19" for short. Outbreaks in Spain and Italy overwhelmed hospital capacity and led to a lockdown of all of Italy. In

Intentionally Infecting Humans. Seema K. Shah, Oxford University Press. © Seema K. Shah 2026.
DOI: 10.1093/9780197667927.003.0005

late February, the US Centers for Disease Control (CDC) announced that serious mitigation efforts, including school closures and the shutting down of businesses, were likely to occur (Centers for Disease Control, 2023). For most people in the United States, however, life proceeded as normal, but with a cloud of uncertainty about what was to come.

The WHO did not declare a public health emergency until March 11, 2020, after more than 100,000 cases and over 4,000 deaths from COVID-19. The Trump administration declared a national emergency 2 days later, and states in the United States began shutting down schools and workplaces. On March 28, 2020, the federal government extended "social distancing measures" through the end of April (Centers for Disease Control, 2023). Initially, because children were at much lower risk than older adults, children were deprioritized in the COVID-19 response (Mintz et al., 2021). On March 31, 2020, it was estimated at a White House Press briefing that 100,000–240,000 people were expected to die in the United States from COVID-19, even if all public health precautions were adopted and implemented—a figure that was shocking at the time (Centers for Disease Control, 2023). As of 2024, more than 1,000,000 people had died due to COVID-19 in the United States (National Center for Health Statistics, 2024), and approximately 14.8 million people lost their lives around the world (Msemburi et al., 2023).

In addition to public health measures such as masking, physical distancing, and limiting large gatherings of people, a major focus of the response to COVID-19 was vaccine development. It was widely believed that if enough people were vaccinated, the world could return to "normalcy" (Higgins-Dunn N, 2020). In early January 2020, a team at the Viral Pathogenesis Lab at the US National Institutes of Health (NIH)'s Vaccine Research Center had begun working on developing a vaccine to combat this new virus. For decades, these researchers had been working on an innovative approach to vaccination that used messenger RNA to instruct the body to produce antibodies against pathogens before they entered host cells, work that was initially fueled by the desire to understand why respiratory syncytial virus (RSV) vaccines had not been successful (Glim, 2021). The US government founded "Operation Warp Speed" and convened several experts who made key decisions about the COVID-19 response, including the decision to create a streamlined approach to testing vaccines that took great financial risks but made it possible to learn about the safety and efficacy of vaccines more rapidly than had ever been done before (Slaoui & Hepburn, 2020).

In the meantime, some quickly latched on to the idea of controlled human infection (CHI) research as a brilliant idea to develop vaccines as quickly as possible (Eyal et al., 2020). The dramatic simplicity of CHI research had broad appeal. As noted in Chapter 4, more academic articles were written about CHI research than ever before (Katzer et al., 2023), not to mention articles in the popular press, publicized debates, and even a TED Talk (Eyal, 2020). A bipartisan group from Congress sent a letter to the NIH urging the consideration and approval of CHI research, and an open letter advocating for CHI research on COVID-19 was signed by celebrities, academics, and even 15 Nobel Prize laureates (Aaronson et al., 2020).

As I demonstrate in this chapter, the excitement over the use of CHI research for COVID-19 suffered from an abundance of hype. The CHI models that were ultimately developed by the United Kingdom did not hasten access to vaccines and have arguably not yielded results that have made a major impact in how COVID-19 is prevented or treated. In light of the history of CHI research and the kinds of contributions from it in the past discussed in Chapter 1, this outcome is less surprising than one might initially think. Nevertheless, the possibility that CHI research could help address emerging infectious diseases in the future remains. This is unlikely to be the last pandemic humans will have to face. For this reason, figuring out *why* CHI research has not (yet) made a major contribution to the response to COVID-19 seems critically important.

Some have argued that the problem for CHI research with SARS-CoV-2 was an excess of precautionary ethics. Without so much deliberation over whether CHI research could be ethical, they argue, CHI research could have made a much bigger difference. There is no doubt that CHI research could be delayed by ethics review; in 2017, a Zika virus CHI model was put on pause due to ethical concerns by a panel chaired by this author (Shah et al., 2018). While the members of the panel felt a cautious approach was warranted, researchers who planned this study objected that the ethics consultation had "slammed the door on progress" (Baumgaertner, 2018).

Does the field of bioethics present the most important obstacle to the use of CHI research for emerging infectious diseases? In this chapter, I explore whether and how CHI research might be best placed to address emerging infectious diseases given the complex and/or unresolved ethical issues it can raise, with special attention to the proposed and actual uses of CHI research in the Zika virus epidemic that began in 2015 and the COVID-19 pandemic. Quite apart from ethics approval, I argue that CHI research has built-in limitations that hold it back from addressing emerging infectious diseases as part of the initial emergency response. I show this by explaining how CHI research during the COVID-19 pandemic failed to live up to the hype for foreseeable reasons. Generally speaking, CHI research is better thought of as a longer-term investment. I argue that, despite the fact that CHI research did not make vaccines for COVID-19 available any sooner, there could be an important, and ethical, role for CHI research as a back-up plan in pandemics that play out differently than the COVID-19 pandemic and in long-term preparations for future pandemics.

Zika Virus

While now overshadowed by the COVID-19 pandemic, in 2015, the Zika virus epidemic was terrifying. Zika virus had been discovered by accident in 1947, in Uganda's Zika forest. Scientists were testing monkeys for yellow fever and discovered another type of flavivirus that they decided to name after the forest in which they found it (Dick et al., 1952). To convey a sense of the isolated nature of the site, in Luganda, a Ugandan language, the term "Zika" means "overgrown" (Shankar, 2019). At that time, it was still not understood how Zika virus affected humans. In 1956, a scientist named William Bearcroft wanted to investigate the potential symptoms associated with this relatively new virus. To that end, he reported deliberately infecting a single 34-year-old European male who volunteered for this rudimentary CHI model (Bearcroft, 1956). Bearcroft was interested in whether this man would have symptoms, such as jaundice, based on prior reports of what Zika could do to the human body, but the research participant experienced nothing more than a fever and a headache. Bearcroft took pains to describe his participant as a "volunteer" but did not address the ethics of his study in any meaningful way—he provided no details about the consent process and failed to indicate whether or how much this volunteer was paid to participate. In 1964, a case report about the clinical course of this illness in a person who was naturally infected was published, also indicating that Zika virus appeared to cause only mild illness (Simpson, 1964).

This early research supported a general belief that Zika virus was not a major public health threat. Very little can be found in the published literature about Zika virus for several decades afterward. Only 14 cases were documented until approximately 2007, when there was an outbreak of Zika virus on the island of Yap in the South Pacific (Duffy et al., 2009). This outbreak similarly did not result in serious illness or deaths, and patients experienced rashes, muscle aches, and conjunctivitis (commonly referred to as "pink eye"). Researchers studying the outbreak after it occurred identified 185 cases suspected to involve Zika virus disease; it was estimated that more than 900 people were infected in less than 3 months. Although they knew that Zika virus was an arbovirus and believed it to be transmitted by mosquitoes, they could not determine how Zika had been transmitted with certainty. The researchers warned that "clinicians and public health officials should be aware of the risk of further expansion of Zika virus transmission" (Duffy et al., 2009).

In 2013–2014, Zika virus spread to other islands in the Pacific Ocean. Studies in French Polynesia found an increase in fetal abnormalities after this outbreak (Cauchemez et al., 2016). It therefore seems that Zika virus may have undergone a mutation that both increased the harm it could cause and its ability to be transmitted, particularly between pregnant individuals and fetuses (Shan et al., 2020). Scientists identified a new condition called *congenital Zika syndrome*, in which fetuses could have microcephaly (abnormal brain development resulting in a head size that is much smaller than normal), with partial collapse of the skull and severe brain damage, damage to the eyes, muscle stiffness that can restrict the body's movement, and many other physical impairments (Melo et al., 2016). It is not possible to know for certain, however, whether Zika mutated over time to cause such devastating effects to a developing fetus or if these sequelae were simply not noticed previously. The serious harm caused by Zika virus to fetuses and young infants is rare enough that it may not have been observed in earlier, smaller outbreaks, and it is possible that not many pregnant people were infected prior to 2015. Furthermore, as a by-product of global injustice, many parts of the world lack the health infrastructure to capture a small increase in serious fetal abnormalities and deaths (Rossi et al., 2018).

In 2015, Zika virus reached Brazil and exploded throughout the country (Rossi et al., 2018). This was when it was first noted that Zika virus was associated with microcephaly in exposed fetuses. Zika virus spread rapidly throughout the Americas, as far North as Canada. The virus was now understood to spread through vectors (e.g., mosquitoes) and sexual activity—a rare virus that could spread through both of these modes of transmission.

Many researchers quickly pivoted to studying Zika virus disease, and, in 2016, researchers who had been collaborating on Dengue virus CHI research developed a protocol for developing a Zika virus CHI model (Shah et al., 2017). Anna Durbin, a researcher at Johns Hopkins University, and two researchers from the NIH—Steve Whitehead and Barney Graham—collaborated on a protocol to develop a Zika virus CHI model that then received funding from the National Institutes of Health (NIH) and the Walter Reed Army Institute of Research, followed by approval from an institutional review board at Johns Hopkins University in 2016. What was public at the time was that the researchers' initial plan was to determine the dose that infected most participants without making them too sick to develop a model with a wide range of potential uses, including learning about Zika virus and accelerating the testing of a Zika vaccine and/or treatments. They also mentioned the possibility of preparing a model to be able to test vaccines and treatments if the epidemic slowed down and made it difficult to test interventions in the field. Ethical concerns arose at the NIH about whether a Zika CHI should be conducted, given the uncertain risks involved (Shah et al., 2017).

In the Fall of 2016, I was invited to chair a multidisciplinary panel asked to determine whether Zika virus CHI could be ethically acceptable and, if so, under what conditions. This panel was convened in October 2016 and met in December 2016. The members of this panel included two obstetrician/gynecologists, a neurologist, one CHI researcher, and several ethicists with expertise in different subfields. We heard evidence from epidemiologists, a regulator at the US Food and Drug Administration (FDA), researchers conducting field trials of Zika vaccines, and researchers conducting CHI studies with pathogens other than Zika virus. When I agreed to chair the panel, I was aware of Christine Grady and Frank Miller's paper on the ethics of challenge studies (Miller & Grady, 2001) and naively thought it would be a simple matter to apply this framework to the case at hand. I soon learned that there were many unanswered questions that would need to be addressed in order to decide whether Zika virus challenge trials were ethically acceptable. The two most difficult involved (1) assessing the social value of the contribution that a Zika virus challenge trial could make to the development of a Zika vaccine and (2) evaluating and justifying risks to third parties who could be infected with Zika virus by research participants (Shah et al., 2018).

Our committee deliberated for 2 months before coming to an agreement that these questions could not be addressed to our satisfaction to warrant allowing the trial to proceed. First, we lacked evidence that a Zika virus challenge trial would speed up or otherwise enhance vaccine development. We had heard from epidemiologists that Zika virus was continuing to spread and likely to remain a threat for years to come. Significantly, we also heard from vaccine developers and clinical trialists that they were working as quickly as possible to test Zika vaccines and had no clear plans to change their approaches based on the results of a Zika CHI study. Second, there was considerable uncertainty about how to prevent harm to third parties outside of the research—an issue that had received scant attention in the bioethics literature. At the time, the CDC advised that people infected with Zika virus might be able to transmit the virus to others for up to 6 months after infection. While confining participants to a hospital or hotel could be one way to prevent them from infecting others, the longest anyone had been confined in CHI research that we could find at the time was about 3 weeks (Shah et al., 2017).

Given that Zika was sexually transmissible, our panel spent some time discussing which groups of people would be least likely to transmit Zika virus to others. One member of our panel suggested that monks and nuns could be enrolled in the study; another darkly responded that there was plenty of evidence that taking a vow of celibacy was no guarantee one would remain celibate. After learning that women were less likely to transmit Zika virus during sexual intercourse than men, we advised that it may be valuable to minimize risk by enrolling only women in the trial and requiring them to use barrier protection and long-acting contraception. Yet we still were worried about chains of transmission, contemplating the possibility of a female being infected with Zika, transmitting it to a sexual partner, and having that sexual partner transmit it to another person who became pregnant. We were skeptical that researchers could monitor participants and ensure they were being careful for 6 months after being infected with Zika virus (Shah et al., 2017).

We initially wrote a lengthy report recognizing the potential merits of doing a challenge study and detailing our concerns, but without making a firm recommendation. After emailing the report to the National Institute of Allergy and Infectious Disease (NIAID) leadership, I was invited to join a call from Anthony Fauci, then director of that institute. In short, Dr. Fauci was not satisfied with the report as written. Dr. Fauci asked for our panel to provide a clear recommendation regarding what to do about the study that the leadership at NIAID could use for their decision-making. Dr. Fauci was also somewhat surprised at our concerns, and he thought that uncertain risks of Zika virus for the participants themselves would have been most concerning to us—including a recent report that Zika virus damaged the testicles of mice (Govero et al., 2016). Our panel met again by teleconference to see if we could coalesce around a clearer recommendation, and I spoke with several members individually to understand their concerns. Some people were concerned that the conclusions were too conservative, asking why we should not allow people to sign up for a high level of risk if they understood what they were getting into. Others had concerns about greenlighting a challenge study with this much uncertainty about the course of the disease and how to prevent its most serious effects for participants. All agreed there remained unanswered questions about the value of the challenge study in light of other research on Zika virus vaccines and the lack of any clear guidance on addressing risks to third parties. We finally reached agreement that it would be premature to conduct the study given these concerns about social value and third-party risk, and we prepared an executive summary to add to the report that stated this view (Shah et al., 2017).

In February 2017, we finally issued our report recommending that Zika CHI research could be ethically justified in principle, provided certain conditions were met, but that those conditions could not be satisfactorily addressed. More specifically, we felt the study should be paused because it was (1) unclear how to mitigate risk to third parties outside of the study, and (2) we had no clear evidence that the studies would help vaccine development (Shah et al., 2017).

It would be an understatement to say the researchers involved in this study were not pleased with this outcome. Two articles came out, one in *STAT News* (Branswell, 2017) and another in *The New York Times*, about the report. Both articles, unfortunately, treated a complex issue as black-and-white, highlighting the disagreement between the ethics panel's recommendation and the researchers. As noted above, the *New York Times* article included the claim that the panel was opposed to scientific progress (Baumgaertner, 2018), and the *STAT News* piece minimized the concerns about third-party risks and highlighted concerns that ongoing vaccine trials would not be able to be completed if the outbreaks continued to wane (Branswell, 2017). An article was also published in a Spanish-language newspaper that made it seem as if a Zika challenge trial was going forward. I subsequently learned that a research participant withdrew from a Zika vaccine study that was being conducted by NIAID—notably not CHI research but simply testing the safety and efficacy of Zika vaccines—because she was afraid she would be infected with Zika virus by the researchers (Eisinger, 2017).

In the summer of 2017, it became clear that Zika field trials could not proceed because outbreaks of the virus had become too sporadic to support them. The WHO, NIH, and FDA collaborated on a meeting that attempted to reach consensus on whether Zika challenge trials could go forward (Vannice et al., 2019). In addition to the compelling case for the need for Zika virus challenge trials, new data emerged showing that people infected with Zika virus were only infectious for

30 days (Paz-Bailey et al., 2018)—a much shorter time period than the 6 months the CDC had indicated was needed to prevent transmission and also a more reasonable length of time to expect participants to remain compliant with precautions against transmission.

Our committee had anticipated that conditions might change and recommended that members of our committee or another body could apply the ethical conditions we had laid out to assess whether a Zika virus CHI model could be ethical to develop in the future (Shah et al., 2017). Although there was no easy way to reconvene the entire committee, at this WHO/NIH/FDA meeting, I shared my view that the need for a Zika virus CHI model to test vaccines meant that the social value of developing a CHI model for Zika virus was high, given that this was now the only viable way to advance a Zika virus vaccine. Additionally, I expressed my view that the fact that participants would only have to take precautions to avoid spreading Zika virus through sexual activity for 1 month (rather than 6 months) was also reassuring and suggested the risks to third parties could be effectively minimized to a low level (Vannice et al., 2019).

Subsequently, the investigators of the trial also requested an ethics consult from their institutional research ethics consultation service at Johns Hopkins, and this ethics consultation report determined that the study could be ethically justified (Karron, 2019). This report is not a public document, and I did not receive permission to share its contents here, but its analysis applied the criteria the panel had laid out for assessing the ethics of creating a Zika virus CHI model and concluded it was now ethically acceptable to proceed. Although it was delayed due to the COVID-19 pandemic, a Zika CHI model has now been developed (Lenharo, 2023; Martinez-Perez et al., 2024). Undoubtedly, the potential use of CHI research for the emerging Zika virus helped raise consciousness about this research method and set the stage for a global debate around the use of CHI research to address COVID-19.

COVID-19

Beginning in late March 2020, several commentators argued that a CHI model with the novel coronavirus (SARS-CoV-2) could bring about a quicker end to the pandemic by hastening vaccine availability (Katzer et al., 2023). Perhaps the first to make this claim were Nir Eyal, Marc Lipsitch, and Peter Smith, who argued as follows: "We believe that controlled SARS-CoV-2 vaccine challenge studies may accelerate the time it takes to evaluate and license vaccines and hence could make vaccines available sooner for widespread rollout" (Eyal et al., 2020). One key argument that they and others made was that, in an emergency like the COVID-19 pandemic, every option should be on the table. For example, Stan Plotkin and Art Caplan wrote a paper advocating for CHI research on COVID-19 that was entitled "Extraordinary Disease Require Extraordinary Solutions" and closed with the following Shakespearean quote: "Desperate diseases by desperate measures are relieved" (Plotkin & Caplan, 2020).

Others, however, raised ethical, logistical, and practical concerns about the use of a SARS-CoV-2 CHI model. Some felt that a treatment was required before CHI research can be ethical (McPartlin et al., 2020). As I argued in Chapter 4, specific treatments are not necessary or sufficient to justify the conduct of CHI research. Rather, the key question is whether the risks in a CHI study are sufficiently understood and are outweighed by the potential benefits. Spinola and colleagues raised concerns about the high degree of uncertainty involved in CHI research (Spinola et al., 2021). Others raised concerns about whether CHI research was indeed likely to be faster than traditional vaccine trials and also highlighted other tradeoffs that could accompany the use of this research method.

For example, I collaborated on a co-authored paper led by Christine Grady in which we argued that the ethical tradeoffs for CHI research did not compare favorably to traditional vaccine trials that were published in August 2020 (Grady et al., 2020). We contended that CHI research for COVID-19 required compromising generalizability because they involved small numbers of people who were at low risk, was not likely to be faster, and also could threaten public trust. It is worth noting that the importance of having the research participants come from diverse backgrounds was critical enough that the Data Monitoring Committee (DMC) overseeing Moderna's Phase III vaccine trials paused enrollment of some groups to draw more from other groups that had been more affected by COVID-19 (Joffe et al., 2021). If even large-scale vaccine trials needed to work on representation, vaccine testing in CHI research would have had serious deficiencies. CHI research had the further limitation that it required isolating, purifying, and manufacturing a strain to use to develop a model, which meant that any CHI model was always lagging behind the latest variant. By November 2020, Kahn and colleagues argued that CHI research on SARS-CoV-2 was unethical because it was unlikely to facilitate vaccine development and raised concerns about public trust and the degree of risk (2020).

Ultimately, advocacy for CHI research did not carry the day in most of the world. Advocates for CHI research had no success in some countries and limited efficacy in the United States. Several countries considered developing a CHI model for SARS-CoV-2 but did not do so. The US NIH developed a protocol and strain of SARS-CoV-2 for use in a CHI model as a back-up plan that was ultimately considered unnecessary (Cornwall, 2020), given how quickly vaccines were being tested in the field during a surge of infections in the United States.

By contrast, even after vaccine rollout began, UK researchers began conducting CHI models in early 2021 (Killingley et al., 2022). The initial CHI models were developed using the strain of SARS-CoV-2 that was circulating in March 2020. The first CHI model, run at the Imperial College London, enrolled individuals who had never been infected with SARS-CoV-2. A second CHI model, conducted at Oxford, exposed individuals who had already been infected with SARS-CoV-2 to the virus again (Rapeport et al., 2021). In both of these trials, participants were unvaccinated because the trials were conducted just prior to vaccine rollout. Subsequent CHI research infecting people with different variants has been conducted (Callaway, 2024). However, a major problem with these subsequent attempts at creating models is that high levels of population immunity are making it difficult to infect volunteers, to the point that the latest published results were not able to find a dose that could infect most people (Jackson et al., 2024). This raises serious questions about whether these models will have much utility in testing future interventions (Callaway, 2024). Rather than rush to a conclusion, however, it is worth examining in depth whether this CHI research was ethically appropriate using the framework laid out in Chapter 4.

Sufficient Social Value

While CHI research can produce many different kinds of social value, most of the ethics literature on CHI research to address COVID-19 focused on using it to replace the final phase of vaccine testing—large-scale field trials conducted to determine whether vaccines work to prevent infection or disease (Eyal et al., 2020). The protocol for the SARS-CoV-2 CHI model also highlighted its potential use in vaccine development as a key reason to create the model. Specifically, the researchers argued that a CHI model was important because "There is significant interest from vaccine producers with novel vaccine candidates not yet in field trials to use the challenge model to quickly determine proof of concept for their vaccine and/or provide supportive efficacy data to apply for emergency licensure of the vaccine" (Killingley et al., 2022). They also attempted to address the counterargument that vaccines could be tested in field studies instead of in a CHI study as follows: "Field trials of all kinds will become increasingly difficult and slow to conduct once widespread vaccination begins and natural infections decrease. Human challenge studies may therefore become the only way to test efficacy for most candidates (with young adults being last and least likely to be vaccinated) and to definitively understand the strength of immune protection quickly enough to make an impact on public health strategy" (Killingley et al., 2022).

Unlike the experience with Zika discussed earlier in this chapter, however, vaccine testing moved forward at an incredibly accelerated pace. By running different phases of the trials in parallel and having the government support this by taking large financial risks to incentivize vaccine manufacturers (but not increase risks to participants), vaccines were developed in record time (Slaoui & Hepburn, 2020). Phase I testing did not wait for animal testing to be concluded; instead, studies were run "in parallel rather than sequentially" to speed up the process. Phase I testing began in March 2020, and the first vaccine was authorized on December 11, 2020.[1] Moderna dosed its first participant on March 16, 2020 (Nedelman, 2020). Pfizer began screening participants for its Phase I/II trial on May 4, 2020 (Mulligan et al., 2020). Results were announced

---

[1] https://www.fda.gov/media/144412/download.

in November 2020 (Bennett, 2020), and the FDA authorized both the Pfizer and Moderna vaccines in December 2020 (Dwyer, 2020). That means that only *7 months* passed for Pfizer's Bio-N-Tech mRNA vaccine from screening participants to emergency use authorization.

Recall that the first CHI model did not begin enrolling until vaccines were already being rolled out. Directly comparing the time it took to set up the CHI model to the time it took to conduct traditional vaccine trials would not seem fair, particularly because some have argued that the ethical debate over CHI research in the COVID-19 pandemic led to excessive delay. Indeed, some scholars suggested that ethical analysis should not focus on biomedical risks of research alone, as the "real risk is excessive caution" (Flanagan, 2021). Similarly, Baay and Neels exhorted as follows: "The longer we wait to set up challenge studies, the lower the chance that they can add valuable information to vaccine development, i.e. add value to regular phase 1–3 trials. The time to act is now" (Baay & Neels, 2020). Eyal and Lipsitch suggested that if a CHI model was developed from the very start of the pandemic by bypassing the need for manufacturing a strain, it could have replaced traditional clinical trials or at least been an important contributor to vaccine research (Eyal & Lipsitch, 2021). As I show below, however, even the argument that CHI research could have contributed much more during COVID-19 is highly unlikely if one considers what is required for the process of developing a CHI model while also keeping in mind the historical and scientific reasons for a cautious approach.

Recall from Chapter 1 that the history of CHI research involves many instances of researchers drawing samples from infectious patients and administering them in challenge studies without knowing exactly what it was they were giving patients. Preparing a strain reliably and safely takes time. Some estimated a CHI strain under Good Manufacturing Processes (GMP) could be prepared in a few weeks or a month (Deming et al., 2020), but many argued it could take as long as a year, and, for the CHI models with SARS-CoV-2 that were conducted, it took approximately 6 months (Killingley et al., 2022). The process of finding the so-called Goldilocks dose took longer. While it is worth considering the possibility of using alternative approaches that may be faster than developing a GMP strain, such as exposing participants to people who have COVID-19 as Eyal and Lipsitch have suggested (Eyal

& Lipsitch, 2021), such an approach would have scientific limitations because it is much harder to control. Before exposing participants to people infected with SARS-CoV-2, it would be important to make sure that the infected patient was only infected with SARS-CoV-2 and nothing else. Additionally, it would be less straightforward to derive what dose of virus participants were given. Standardizing the approach to get a consistent dose of SARS-CoV-2 would likely take time, even if it would take less than 6 months. Finally, different people can have large variation in how easily they might become infected and/or infect others in ways that are hard to predict and not tied to the severity of their symptoms; something that was, somewhat ironically, shown by the SARS-CoV-2 CHI models (Killingley et al., 2022). Therefore, it might have taken at least 6 months to standardize a "natural infection" model and could likely have been very difficult to do, if not impossible.

Perhaps the more "artificial" version of the model could have been developed more quickly and thereby contributed to the acceleration of vaccine research. Unfortunately, comparing the time it took to conduct the first UK CHI model once it was started to the time it took to test vaccines in a more traditional way reveals that this was also unlikely.

For the United Kingdom's first CHI model, the Health Research Ethics Committee approved a screening protocol on December 2, 2020. To save time, the research team immediately began screening potential volunteers. The final protocol was approved in February 2021. The researchers were lucky in that the initial dose they selected was sufficient to infect most participants and not make them too sick—so there was no need to try higher doses in a stepwise fashion (which is often the case for CHI models). Yet it took 7 months simply for all participants to be screened, enrolled, and followed through the initial quarantine period—after final approval was given on February 16, 2021, the first volunteers were enrolled on March 6, and the last participant left quarantine on July 8, 2021 (Williams et al., 2022; Killingley et al., 2022).

Disseminating the results to an international audience took much longer. The first results were published in a preprint in February 2022 (Killingley et al., 2022) and in final form on March 31, 2022 (Killingley et al., 2022). Notably, these results were from a CHI model, which would then later have to be used to test vaccines. As noted above, the process of creating the model itself took approximately 7 months, not counting the time required for initial approval, aggregation of the findings, cleaning the data, and preparing it for reporting and submission. Recall that, to accelerate vaccine testing, the model would have to then be used in a study where participants are randomized to receive the vaccine or a placebo, which takes several months on top of the time to create the model.

That means that 7 months passed for Pfizer's Bio-N-Tech mRNA vaccine from screening participants to emergency use authorization; this was the *same* amount of time that it took simply from approval of the UK CHI model screening protocol through to the completion of enrollment (Figure 5.1).

Admittedly, one factor that made vaccine field testing proceed so quickly was the uncontrolled nature of the COVID-19 epidemic in the United States at the time testing occurred (Joffe et al., 2021). The fact that so many people in the trials were naturally becoming infected with COVID made the trials reach their endpoints faster. This suggests that if COVID had been more like Zika—easier to control in the short run but still posing a significant threat in the long run—a CHI model may have been useful because traditional vaccine trials might have failed to determine whether vaccines were efficacious. Additionally, if strict public health measures such as masking and physical distancing had been more feasible all over the world (as was the case in New Zealand and Australia for some time and was the case in China for even longer), a CHI model might have been the only way to move

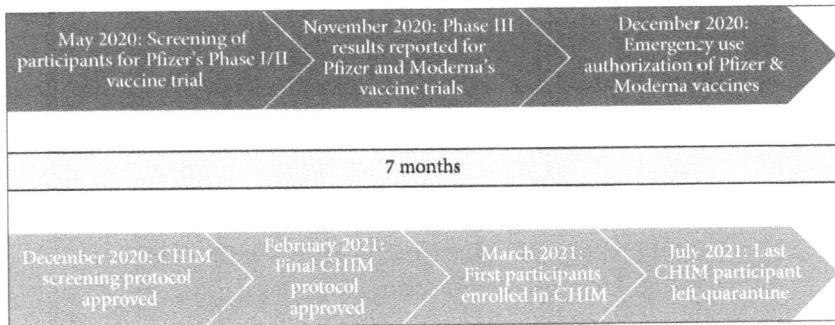

Figure 5.1 Comparison of timeline for vaccine trials versus SARS-CoV-2 controlled human infection (CHI) model.

vaccine development along while such public health measures were in place and transmission was occurring very rarely. Yet given the harms associated with strict public health measures (Geulayov et al., 2022) and the erosion of trust in governments and scientific authority during COVID-19 (Kennedy et al., 2022), it seems unlikely that strict public health measures will be implemented successfully all over the world during the next pandemic. Additionally, it is important to recall that there are counterfactuals to consider for CHI models as well. For example, if CHI model researchers had begun with a dose that was much lower and that required escalation to find the right dose, or that was much higher and raised serious safety concerns, the process of creating the model could have taken longer than it did.

While efforts to speed up the creation of CHI models remain important, it is hard to imagine a counterfactual world where a CHI model for SARS-CoV-2 would have been a better option than accelerating traditional clinical trials. Advocates who argued for the brilliant simplicity of CHI research failed to recognize the time it takes to do rigorous CHI research and also did not account for the possibility that traditional vaccine research could be accelerated without compromising safety as long as enough money could be thrown at the problem. Furthermore, speed is not the only relevant criterion in assessing the most appropriate research method. I have argued with others that vaccine trials in the field offer several advantages over testing vaccines in CHI models, including increased generalizability, diversity, larger numbers of participants, and fewer concerns about public trust (Grady et al., 2020).

Although the SARS-CoV-2 CHI models did not accelerate the development of the initial vaccines to address COVID-19, and there is reason to think that their potential to do so was always limited, it is still worth examining what these models have offered in terms of social value.

Sufficient Social Value from the UK SARS-CoV-2 CHI models?

Results from the first two SARS-CoV-2 CHI models with the March 2020 strain provide a strong basis for establishing the safety of the model to enable future use, along with several insights about the virus. Perhaps the most surprising finding from the study was that researchers used a much lower dose of the virus than anyone thought would be necessary to create the model (Killingley et al., 2022). In other words, it was much easier to infect people with no prior immunity from infections or vaccines than experts had anticipated. Recall that to set up a CHI model, researchers need to find the "Goldilocks" dose of the pathogen—the amount that will reliably infect most of the participants (50–70%) without making them too sick. Giving participants very high doses would reliably infect everyone but could end up making the participants very ill. Taking a cautious approach, the researchers started with a dose that was 10 times lower than what the WHO's technical working group had recommended for setting up a CHI model with SARS-CoV-2 (Research & Development Blueprint Team, 2020). As conservative as this initially seemed, it turned out that this dose was the one they were seeking. It was sufficient to infect more than half of the participants—specifically, 18 people out of 34. Moreover, the researchers were using the strain that was circulating in March 2020, which was far less transmissible than later variants (Carabelli et al., 2023). This demonstrates that there is a great deal of uncertainty inherent in creating any new model, particularly one with an emerging infectious disease where little is known about it and the population does not have preexisting immunity.

To further illustrate this uncertainty, recall that there were two models initially developed with the March 2020 strain—one with people who had never been infected with SARS-CoV-2 and another with participants who had been previously infected. Based on the results reported to date, the model with people who had never been infected does appear to have been safe enough for future use. While the researchers did not report any serious harm to the participants, such as hospitalizations or death, a few people lost their senses of smell and taste and one had this persist for months (Killingley et al., 2022). It has not been reported that the participants suffered from the other kinds of harm that have been recognized as being caused by COVID, including damage to the brain and the heart. However, the attempt to develop a model in people who were previously infected was not successful in identifying a dose that could infect most of the people (Jackson et al., 2024).

Other insights from the model with people who had not been infected previously largely confirmed information about COVID that had been learned in other ways by the time the data were published. For example, participants started showing symptoms 2–4 days after they were exposed to the pathogen. Approximately 40 hours after exposure, the throat was the first place that researchers found the virus in participants they had infected, but then it moved to the nose. Viral loads peaked at 5 days. The virus could be found in the nose for a median of 10 days, but for up to 12 days in some people. The implication of this finding reported by the researchers was that it confirmed the importance of wearing masks that cover the nose in addition to the mouth. The study found that people who were asymptomatic often had very high viral loads. Most participants who became infected temporarily lost their senses of smell and taste. One person still had significant loss of smell 180 days after infection, although it was reported to have been improving both by objective measures and the participant's own perception (Killingley et al., 2022).

Researchers also found that much of the important immunity against the virus was concentrated in the nose, along with very high viral shedding (or release of infectious particles into the environment)—more specifically, in and from the nasal passages. As noted above, they also discovered that it was relatively easy to infect people who lacked immunity from vaccines or previous infections but much more difficult to infect people who had been previously infected (Jackson et al., 2023). Participants also became infectious within 24–48 hours. This was suggested by previous epidemiological data but answered more definitively by the CHI model. When previous studies had observed how quickly people were able to infect others, one limitation was that people could have had multiple exposures, and it was difficult to rule out that possibility. The SARS-CoV-2 CHI model had a distinct advantage: researchers could control the variables to ensure that only one exposure happened, and the amount of virus a person started shedding could be measured very precisely. This also enabled them to show that there are dramatic differences between how infectious different people are without necessarily determining the source of these differences (Zhou et al., 2023), though other studies also revealed similar differences in infectiousness among different people that led to the use of the term "superspreaders" for people who were highly infectious (Edwards et al., 2021).

Additionally, the SARS-CoV-2 CHI model showed that *lateral flow testing* (also referred to as *rapid antigen testing*, which is available in at-home test kits that reveal whether someone is infected with the virus in 30 minutes or less) is highly effective at catching whether someone was infected if the test is repeated over the course of a few days (Zhou et al., 2023). Some have argued that this finding changed policy and practice in the United Kingdom by allowing the country to come out of lockdown sooner through confirming that a strategy of repeated use of at-home tests after exposure would help people identify infection early and prevent them from unwittingly infecting others (World Health Organization Roundtable, 2024).

There have been additional publications reporting other results from the UK CHI models. One article reported findings about the presence of virus in the air and in the environment after exposure to SARS-CoV-2 (Zhou et al., 2023). This study found wide variation on when, how, and how much virus was emitted by different people, including that those who had the most symptoms did not necessarily spread the most virus. The study authors noted that they found "two of the 18 infected participants emitting a large proportion (approximately 90%) of airborne virus on just 1 or 2 days" (Zhou et al., 2023). They also found virus on small surfaces that were frequently touched (e.g., doorknobs), on larger surfaces, and on participants' hands.

Interestingly, the article includes a box summarizing other similar studies and what this research added to what was known at the time. It notes that there have been studies examining the presence of SARS-CoV-2 in the air and on surfaces in hospitals, and that one study recruited infected participants a few days into the course and conducted a similar analysis of the virus that they shed. The authors point out that the rigor and precision with which a CHI model could address these questions is clearly an improvement over other types of research (Zhou et al., 2023). What remains unclear, however, is whether that precision had enough utility to justify conducting a CHI model. The implications the authors themselves present suggest that it may have been the latter. By August 2023, most people open to scientific evidence already knew the implications the authors highlighted (i.e., that it is important to wear masks over the nose and not just the mouth, that hand hygiene and indoor surface cleaning are important in addition to addressing possible airborne transmission, and that rapid testing can help identify when people are contagious). The authors also noted that their findings suggest that blocking transmission with antiviral nasal sprays is a promising strategy, which may be less widely known, but intranasal vaccines have been in development and testing for some time (Shapira et al., 2022).

Another paper highlighted an interesting finding that people infected with SARS-CoV-2 scored significantly worse on cognitive tests compared to a control group that was not infected, particularly related to executive functioning and memory, although the differences were relatively small. These findings persisted for a year after infection. These results are particularly interesting because all participants had mild (or no) symptoms, and did not report that they felt there was any change in their cognitive function. The authors noted that the results from this study confirmed other research showing a decline in cognitive scores after infection with SARS-CoV-2, but were able to do so more rigorously because of the detailed knowledge of when people were infected in the CHI model and what their course of illness was like (Trender et al., 2024).

The researchers have also published an abstract indicating that they have identified a correlate of protection when trying to develop a SARS-CoV-2 CHI model (Jackson et al., 2023). In a CHI model with people who had previously been infected with the virus, the investigators reported that they increased the dose of the virus repeatedly but were only able to infect 5 out of 36 people who had prior infection, using a relatively high dose. They found that those who were able to be reinfected had lower levels of antibodies to SARS-CoV-2 in the mucosa of the nose and throughout the body in addition to lower levels of interferon-gamma, which is a cytokine that plays an important role in the immune response. Identifying correlates of protection can be very useful for many reasons. For example, correlates of protection can serve as surrogate markers that can be used to test new vaccines and determine whether they offer protection without having to wait to see a difference in those who become infected and those who do not across a vaccine and placebo arm. The authors note in this abstract, however, that these correlates of protection need further testing and validation, suggesting that the value from this insight might be incremental and not definitive.

Reviewing these data suggests that the social value of the first UK CHI models with SARS-CoV-2 was not compelling. In particular, it is unclear whether there was high social value from developing a SARS-CoV-2 CHI model with people who had not had COVID-19 just before the rollout of vaccines. Admittedly, the risks associated with creating a CHI model evolved over the course of the pandemic. Once effective vaccines and treatments for COVID-19 were available, and large numbers of people had some level of preexisting immunity from vaccines or prior infections, the risk associated with CHI research was reduced, which in turn decreased the burden of justification for developing a CHI model. This suggests that, as long as something valuable could be learned from a CHI model, they became easier to justify over the course of the pandemic, and particularly so after more people were vaccinated and better treatments emerged. Thus, later models may have had enough social value to justify the risk, even if the first model did not. Yet later models have so far found it difficult to identify doses that can infect most people now that there is a high level of population immunity from vaccines and previous infections, limiting their value in another important way.

Information was also slow to be published from the UK CHI models, which further limited their social value. In meetings involving interested parties, it has been suggested that the UK government received early findings from the CHI models that informed the pandemic response and also that the involvement of government actors slowed the process of disseminating information publicly (World Health Organization Roundtable, 2024). These claims are plausible, if difficult to verify, but would also suggest that what social value these models produced was concentrated in the UK and not broadly shared.

While it is challenging to assess the social value of creating a new CHI model with SARS-CoV-2 because of the possibility that these models could be used in other ways in the future, another limitation of these models is their diminished relevance over time. Insights related to the early strains may not translate to future strains. Because CHI models are always playing catch-up to an ever-evolving virus, they may reveal insights that have decreased value over time. The fact that recent CHI models have struggled to find a dose that is high enough to affect participants raises doubts about these prospects (Callaway, 2024). Finally, there may be alternative ways to learn similar information. As was demonstrated throughout the COVID-19 pandemic and will be discussed further below, creative study designs can answer many scientific questions without deliberately infecting anyone with a pathogen.

Addressing COVID-19 with Alternatives to CHI Research

The results from the UK CHI model that have been described as the most important to date are the insights into the pathogen itself. While it is true that CHI research can more carefully and precisely study a pathogen to learn insights that can be difficult to learn in other ways, researchers have a number of methods at their disposal to answer questions about a new pathogen.

One important way to study SARS-CoV-2 is through animal models. This includes the creation of humanized mouse models and non-human primate models, like rhesus macaques. During the COVID-19 pandemic, an infection challenge study was conducted with rhesus macaques to test Moderna's mRNA-1273 vaccine (DeGrazia & Miller, 2021). This study was conducted at the same time that Phase I studies with human volunteers began, rather than being done beforehand, which is the standard way that animal trials involving vaccines for human use are usually done. Conducting animal studies in parallel with human testing was one way of speeding up the process of vaccine development. An ethical analysis of this nonhuman animal challenge trial found that the general justification for the trial appeared to be on solid ground, because if there had been safety or efficacy concerns emerging from this trial, they could have been incorporated into decisions about whether to proceed with later phases of trials with this vaccine. However, the authors did raise concerns about the potential for unnecessary harm in this study. For instance, the animals in the trial were killed at the end of it to allow examination of the monkeys' lungs to look for evidence that they had experienced severe disease. They did not find any such evidence in vaccinated monkeys, but it also is unclear that such information was necessary to decide whether vaccines were promising enough to move on to further testing (DeGrazia & Miller, 2021). Additionally, animal models have some limitations, and the systemic inflammatory response gone awry that is seen in some humans with COVID-19 does not seem to occur in non-human primates, suggesting that the model may have been more useful for investigating mild cases of COVID-19 rather than revealing information about protection from severe disease (Harrison et al. 2020).

There are also many ways to approach research with human subjects that revealed insights about SARS-CoV-2 (Harrison et al., 2020). For example, air sampling studies can test the amount of the virus circulating in the air (Comber et al., 2021). Studies of coronaviruses related to SARS-CoV-2 have helped illuminate several aspects of the disease and how it is transmitted, including that there can be transmission through respiratory droplets, aerosol, direct contact with contaminated surfaces, and by ingesting food contaminated with fecal particles (Yu et al., 2004). Modeling studies have been used to estimate the amount of spread of the virus from people who are infected but do not yet exhibit any symptoms (Harrison et al., 2020). Case studies can provide information about what happened to individual patients, and observational studies can provide clues about why some people become infected and not others.

For one example of how different kinds of research can be put together to learn about transmission, an observational study of COVID-19 patients in China found that daily eyeglass wearers were less often infected with SARS-CoV-2 than the general population (Zeng et al., 2020). Deng and Bao later conducted an experimental study successfully infecting rhesus macaques through the eye (or, more specifically, conjunctiva), suggesting that this might be a way that humans can be infected with SARS-CoV-2 as well (Deng et al., 2020). This has led to the recommendation that goggles or other eye protection can help prevent transmission of SARS-CoV-2 (Szczęśniak & Brydak-Godowska, 2021).

As another example, a study was conducted at the University of Illinois at Urbana-Champaign to better understand transmission of SARS-CoV-2. This study took advantage of the requirement that faculty, staff, and students had polymerase chain reaction (PCR) testing for SARS-CoV-2 at least twice a week. The study team enrolled people who had symptoms, who remained symptom-free, and who started off symptom-free and later developed symptoms. They recruited people who had a negative test in the previous 7 days and then a positive test within 24 hours or were 5 days post-exposure to someone who had tested positive, which enabled them to catch people in the very early days of infection. They collected nasal and saliva samples for 14 days and asked people to fill out a daily survey of their symptoms. Most of the people in this study were young, non-Hispanic white, and male, so the data suffered a little from the same generalizability problem seen in CHI research. Nevertheless, this study found that there was a great deal of variability between how the virus moved throughout the bodies of individuals. They found 9 out of 60 people had no virus in their nasal swabs even though they were infected. The study team found that participants were more likely to test positive on viral culture on days when they had muscle aches, a runny nose, and a scratchy throat—suggesting that those symptoms are associated with being more infectious. While they found that, for most people, the peak time when they were shedding virus in saliva was 1 day prior to when the virus could be found from nasal swabs, for four participants, the reverse was true. Moreover, the study team found that the differences in people's infectiousness were not fully explained by how much of the virus could be detected—there seem to be other things going on, such as variation among the people themselves or their environments. Increasing age was also associated with greater infectiousness. The study team was also able to compare the B.1.1.7 strain to the original strain of COVID and found no major differences in terms of the release of viral particles into the environment from infected people (Ke et al., 2022).

Another approach has been to use the examination of tissues by pathologists (including tissues derived by conducting autopsies of the bodies of deceased COVID patients) with sophisticated laboratory techniques. Scientists can thereby put together information learned by studying tissues under a microscope with data on cell types and their patterns of expression. Lab testing can model what happens as the virus moves into different cells in different parts of the body. This type of work, combined with data from the original SARS-CoV-1, has shown that specific cells in the nose, throat, and airway are likely to be the first cells targeted during infection (Lamers & Haagmans, 2022).

To be fair, it is possible that the level of rigor and depth with which COVID CHI models can study early disease and transmission has no true alternative. Yet it is not immediately obvious that this level of rigor and depth is of high value. There is certainly intrinsic value in science and discovery that broadens human understanding. Additionally, the role of serendipity in science has revealed the value of learning information that could be useful in ways we cannot yet anticipate. However, claims about potential social value because of additional precision are likely unable to bear the weight of justification for research with high and uncertain long-term risks. This suggests that the deliberate infection of participants with the March 2020 strain of SARS-CoV-2 just prior to vaccination likely did not have sufficient social value.

While there were alternative ways to find many of the same things that were discovered by the UK researchers, CHI models may continue to be useful to test things that are hard to study in other ways, provided that models can be set up with newer variants for which it is still possible to induce infection—which is an open question (Callaway, 2024). For example, CHI studies could help answer open questions about treatments, such as what an optimal dose might be. CHI studies could be very useful in continuing to refine correlates of protection or fast-tracking new diagnostic tests for COVID-19 (Edwards & Neuzil, 2022). Finally, some have suggested CHI research is best thought of as an "accelerant" for research, promoting quick failures of some candidate interventions and prioritizing others for future study. CHI studies are used in malaria research in just this way. CHI research is rarely a self-contained approach to testing new products. However, future CHI studies could be one step in a larger process that makes the entire process go faster. By helping to prioritize which vaccines or treatments are the most promising, researchers can select interventions for future testing. This could be important because if people have already been vaccinated and/or infected with COVID-19 multiple times, the trials that will be conducted may need larger numbers of people and more time to be able to see whether the interventions make a difference in protecting people against infection or ameliorating symptoms short of severe disease—provided of course that new models can be created. Importantly, however, it is not clear that the models created earlier in the COVID-19 pandemic were necessary to create models with newer variants today, again casting doubt on the justification for developing those early models in the first place.

Did the UK CHI models Have a Reasonable Risk–Benefit Ratio?

As discussed above, the original SARS-CoV-2 CHI models were created in the United Kingdome in December 2021. The risks posed by a SARS-CoV-2 CHI model were systematically analyzed by another researcher who was considering conducting a CHI model, Meta Roestenberg, and several colleagues in November 2020 (Kuiper et al., 2021). This analysis provides a helpful snapshot of what was known and not known about COVID-19 at that time, roughly at the same time as the first protocol was submitted to the UK Health Research Authority.

For participants, Roestenberg and colleagues focused on the risks that they would experience severe disease, antibody-dependent enhancement (i.e., the theoretical risk that people who were infected with COVID could have more severe cases if they are infected again later), long COVID, and negative effects from being isolated from others. They also raised the risks of transmission to others in the community. This list of potential risks is comprehensive, with the main omission being the potential for the risk of a loss of public trust if a participant in a CHI model was seriously injured or if they infected someone else outside of the research.

In this analysis, Roestenberg and colleagues found a low risk of severe outcomes based on the available data and assumptions that a population at low risk from serious complications would be enrolled in the study. They assumed that people under the age of 30 without known comorbidities that could increase the severity of COVID would be enrolled in the CHI model, which was the case in the UK CHI models. With that assumption in place, they argued that the available data suggested that there would be between a very low rate of death

(1.2–6.1 deaths per 100,000 infections). They further argued that this was lower than the road deaths in that age group in several European countries, suggesting that the risk of severe outcomes in a SARS-CoV-2 CHI model was comparable to the risks of daily life. The protocol that was ultimately used in the UK CHI models indeed included an extensive list of exclusion criteria, as contemplated by Roestenberg and colleagues, that included obesity and comorbidities such as kidney disease and diabetes. The researchers also used the QCovid tool that had been developed in the United Kingdom to identify how high a risk of severe disease or death individuals faced, and they excluded participants who had a risk score that crossed a prespecified threshold (Killingley et al., 2022).

To mitigate the risks of severe disease and death, Roestenberg and colleagues further proposed the use of several treatments, such as remdesivir, dexamethasone, and potentially convalescent plasma and monoclonal antibodies. While treatment is not required for a CHI model to be ethical depending on whether there are other ways to mitigate risk, the only treatments for COVID-19 available at this time that had evidence of effectiveness were remdesivir and monoclonal antibodies. The researchers began by giving what they called "pre-emptive" remdesivir before the onset of serious symptoms, but discontinued this once the Data and Safety Monitoring Board and Trial Steering Committee determined this was not needed to protect participants. There was a plan to provide monoclonal antibodies to participants if they met prespecified "clinical severity criteria," but no participants did, so monoclonal antibodies were not used (Killingley et al., 2022).

With respect to the risk of antibody-dependent enhancement (or that participants might have more severe disease if they had previously been infected or vaccinated), Roestenberg and colleagues felt this risk was still theoretical and therefore of a low probability. Based on this theoretical risk, however, they recommended not conducting CHI models with people who had been previously infected with SARS-CoV-2, although this was one of the models tested in the United Kingdom. While risks should generally be assessed *ex ante*, we now know that antibody-dependent enhancement is not likely to be an issue (Gan et al., 2022). In fact, prior infection with SARS-CoV-2 protects against future infection for some period of time (Havervall et al., 2022).

The risk of long COVID was also important to consider, although this risk was highly uncertain because long COVID was poorly understood at that time (and remains incompletely understood now). Roestenberg and colleagues assumed that long COVID was more likely in older people, people with comorbidities, and people who experienced severe disease, so the steps that would be taken to minimize the risks of severe disease would also minimize the risks of long COVID. Ultimately, the SARS-CoV-2 CHI models did report some extended loss of taste and smell among participants but not other long-lasting symptoms. Long COVID has been associated with some symptoms that were likely to manifest within the trial period, such as fatigue, breathlessness, cognitive impairment, trouble with sleep, and headaches (Crook et al., 2021), and others that may yet be less well understood. The initial SARS-CoV-2 CHI model was designed with 1 year of follow-up about loss of smell and any neurological impairment (Killingley et al., 2022).

Regarding negative effects from isolation, Roestenberg and colleagues felt that 2 weeks would be sufficient to ensure protection of third parties, a length of time that is not unprecedented for confinement in CHI research. They suggested ways to mitigate this risk to an acceptable level, such as testing participants frequently and allowing them to leave isolation when they tested negative, as well as providing sufficient compensation to offset the potential loss of income.

The researchers who conducted the CHI model also identified other more minor risks in the protocol, including potential reactivation of herpes virus for participants who had previously had a herpes infection and transient increases in liver enzymes, and they planned to inform participants of these risks, ask about risk factors in advance, and monitor liver enzymes throughout the study.

Another risk was that participants might not receive prompt treatment for any research-related injuries, including longer-term symptoms of SARS-CoV-2 infection. The research team did track participant symptoms for 1 year after enrollment. Additionally, the fact that the model was developed in the United Kingdom was fortunate, as will be relevant to site selection. The UK National Health Service ensured participants would have access to healthcare if they needed in the future—an important protection that research in many countries, including the United States, simply does not have to offer.

In addition to risks to participants, the risk to third parties were also important to consider. With a length of isolation that would cover the infectious period and the use of personal protective equipment for research personnel, Roestenberg and colleagues argued that the risk of community transmission could be minimized substantially with a period of isolation and confinement and would therefore not raise concern. The researchers who designed the UK CHI model also used intranasal drops placed in participants' nostrils rather than aerosolized sprays, which might have more closely mirrored how people become infected outside of the laboratory, to minimize the risk of spreading the virus to research staff. Another risk to consider is that to the public's trust in research. While there has been no formal assessment that I am aware of about whether the UK CHI models had an impact on public trust, the long-term community engagement around CHI models in the UK may have mitigated this risk (Piggin et al., 2022).

While the risks associated with the COVID CHI models that have been reported to date do not appear to be very high, it is not entirely clear whether the risks associated with long COVID have been fully characterized. Additionally, research risks should be assessed *ex ante*, instead of after the fact. Risks related to long COVID and antibody-dependent enhancement were not well-understood at the time these trials were conducted, and the treatment options for preventing these outcomes were limited. The fact that the first CHI models were done after vaccines were being rolled out limited their social value, which suggests that there was not enough social value to justify the risk that these initial CHI models posed. However, CHI research conducted with later strains of SARS-CoV-2, particularly after effective treatment was available and the risk of being infected with the virus really became a part of everyday life, is easier to justify. As of 2024, one could argue that the risk of having COVID-19 is a risk of daily life that would fall under the definition of minimal risk. Indeed, the risk of infection with SARS-CoV-2 is something that most people assume and trade-off against all other types of goods. Attending an academic conference, sporting event, or concert might be worth this risk for some people, but not for others. This suggests it is reasonable to conduct CHI research with SARS-CoV-2 for a broader range of potential societal benefits that may not be substantial but are high enough to justify exposing participants to minimal risk. This research might involve participants who had some prior immunity, whether through vaccination or infection or both, but this would arguably make the model more relevant for testing future interventions.

In sum, it is not clear whether the risks associated with the first two CHI models conducted in the United Kingdom could be justified by the limited social value that was associated with the models to date, but, as the risk level went down over time, CHI models with newer strains of SARS-CoV-2 became easier to justify—while also being much more difficult to conduct successfully.

Suitable Site Selection

As noted in Chapter 4, there are several factors to consider in selecting a site for CHI research. The ethical considerations for site selection include: (1) how much experience the site has with conducting CHI models in general and with CHI models that use the particular type of pathogen, (2) whether there is a robust healthcare system to ensure participants can receive treatment for any longer-term effects of being infected with the pathogen, (3) whether the public health infrastructure can prevent transmission of pathogens or create additional protections if participants withdraw from the study early while infectious, (4) how sensitized the community has been to the concept of research in general and CHI research in particular, (5) whether there is experience at the site in treating the particular pathogen that participants will be infected with, (6) the level of risk of burdening an overburdened healthcare system if CHI research participants become very sick, and (7) the existence of a solid research ethics oversight system that can provide rigorous review of the protocol.

The UK CHI models did relatively well on these criteria. The CHI models were conducted at a high-containment quarantine facility (Rapeport et al., 2021) in a country with a robust healthcare system, public health infrastructure, and research ethics oversight (which was bolstered further, as will be discussed with respect to independent review). Community engagement efforts will be discussed under procedural criteria below, but efforts to sensitize the community to CHI research had been ongoing in the United Kingdom for several years, particularly led by the Human Infection Challenge Study Vaccine (HIC-Vac) network (Barnes et al., 2023).

Notably, taking into light concerns about long COVID from the deliberate infection of participants in CHI research, it may have been ethically preferable to conduct these studies in the United Kingdom rather than the United States. One great failure of American research policy is the lack of a system for compensating injured research participants. Coupled with the lack of a universal healthcare system, the outcome of this policy failure is that participants who have long-term injuries may suffer catastrophic loss of income and support. Accordingly, one critical moral difference between doing the studies in the United States and the United Kingdom is that the United Kingdom has a national health service (and a better social safety net) that could provide care for any participants in CHI research who suffer from long COVID and have chronic complications from their infection. In the absence of a specific plan to compensate and care for injured research participants, this difference alone is a reason that CHI research with infectious agents that have the potential to cause longer-term complications is more ethically problematic in countries that lack universal healthcare, such as the United States, than in countries that provide it.

Fair Participant Selection

In the context of CHI models, Chapter 4 established that fair participant selection should focus on the fair sharing of burdens and risks, including the distribution of third-party risks. As noted above, the UK CHI models involved an effort to reduce risks that excluded participants with obesity and several comorbidities known to increase risk of serious complications from infection. The use of the QCovid tool to further identify risk and the exclusion of participants at higher risk under this algorithm was also important (Killingley, et al., 2022). Finally, the focus on minimizing third-party risks with a longer period of confinement than was thought to be necessary limited the risk to such a low level that the distribution of those risks was not a major concern.

One concern the researchers recognized was that the QCovid score for minoritized groups was typically higher than for people identifying as white, which meant that the QCovid score could limit the diversity of participants. Given that early models with small numbers of people would not be able to reflect the target population no matter what, the decision was made to use the score early in the process but not once the model was proved to be safe (Rapeport et al., 2021), which was a reasonable way to address fairness in selecting participants.

Informed Consent in the UK SARS-CoV-2 CHI models

The informed consent process seemed to be a focal point for the review committee overseeing these studies. The review committee required that information be presented to potential participants, followed by a break to give people an opportunity to think about involvement in the trials and to ask any questions they had. After that point, participants were given a test of understanding of the key facts about the trial that they had to pass before signing a form to authorize their participation. (Davies, 2023). As described, this process generally follows best practices to enhance understanding by giving people time to digest the information and testing their understanding prior to admitting them into the study (Grady et al., 2017).

The participant information sheet for the CHI model using the Delta variant is available online, along with a video about human challenge trials (Imperial College London, 2023). While developing a video is a good idea, this video was merely a voice-over of a PowerPoint presentation that presents the information from the consent document, with only a few pictures and even less intonation. By contrast, this information sheet was very well-designed, with a two-page overview to start and a longer document that could serve as a resource for participants throughout the study.

This information sheet began by laying out the purpose of the CHI model as understanding three things: "how well the Delta

SARS-CoV-2 variant infects previously vaccinated people; what levels of immunity mean people are less likely to get infected; and what happens in 'breakthrough' infection with Delta." It then stated that the study will "pave the way" to test vaccines and treatments for better control of the pandemic. There was "key information" specifically called out for participants, including the following: that participants will be given SARS-CoV-2 virus, that they may lose their sense of smell and taste, that there are small risks of serious injury, and that the study will provide care and has insurance to cover long-term problems participants may have. Much to the research team's credit, it was clearly and explicitly stated in the document that, "If you take part, you will be deliberately given SARS-CoV-2 and may develop COVID-19."

The information sheet also contained a paragraph delineating the risks seen in the initial CHI model created from the virus that was circulating in March 2020, which included that one participant had loss of smell and taste for 9 months that finally resolved by the end of the study. It noted a lesser-appreciated risk of SARS-CoV-2 infection, which included small decreases in memory and cognition for some people. Finally, the sheet addressed the risk of long COVID and notes that, for the group being enrolled (healthy, vaccinated adults between the ages of 18 and 30 years), the risk was approximately 1–2.5%.

Risks to third parties were also tackled head-on. The sheet explained that, for any participants who want to withdraw early, "we will talk to you again in detail about the importance of remaining in the quarantine unit until you are no longer contagious. This is for both your safety and that of others." Relatedly, there was a somewhat unusual addition to this consent form—a code of responsibilities for participants. The first item on the list asked participants to "answer questions about your medical history honestly and completely"—addressing a key concern that the desire to earn money through the study will lead participants to withhold disqualifying information. The code of responsibilities also asked participants to share any symptoms they had with study staff. The code of responsibilities was fairly comprehensive. In a passage that might take older readers back to university life, they also asked participants to keep their inpatient rooms tidy and avoid playing loud music.

There is much to commend about this informed consent process. It was carefully and thoughtfully designed, addressing concerns raised by ethicists and incorporating data-driven practices for informed consent. Perhaps the only major drawback is that the consent form failed to make clear that these CHI models might not be useful for vaccine testing. Our preliminary data have showed that people who signed up on a registry for these trials—notably not those who went through a formal consent process—typically thought their involvement would speed up vaccine development. Some seemed to think that they would receive the vaccine in the CHI model and did not appear to understand the distinction between a CHI model and CHI study. If these participants did not understand that the goal was to develop a model of deliberate infection, and that this model was unlikely to be useful in testing vaccines, the consent process may not have been as robust as it should have been.

Proportionate Payment

The UK CHI models described giving participants a "donation" of up to £4,565 for their time and inconvenience, noting that they were quarantined for at least 17 days. This amount was calculated based on the national living wage in the United Kingdom (Killingley et al., 2022). Although this amount seems relatively high, it is notable that participants were not paid for risk, as some have suggested they should be (Grimwade et al., 2020). Rather, they were paid according to standard accounts of how to compensate participants for the time they spend doing "unskilled" but essential labor (Dickert & Grady, 1999). Participants were also provided with care throughout the study and guaranteed care after the study because of the United Kingdom's national health service, suggesting that they would receive some form of compensation for research-related injury if it were to occur (Lynch et al., 2021). It is unclear whether the study team obtained compensation for other forms of injury, such as long-term disability insurance, although it does not seem that participants would have needed this in the end.

Independent Review

As noted in Chapter 4, the WHO's key criteria for the ethical acceptability of COVID-19 CHI research was released in May 2020 and set out both substantive and procedural criteria for this research, including the use of a specialized independent committee with the relevant expertise to review these studies (Barnes et al., 2023). The UK National Health Service Health Research Authority formed an ad hoc committee specifically to review applications for SARS-CoV-2 CHI research. There were both expert and lay members on this committee. Some of the members had prior experience reviewing CHI research, while others deliberately did not in order to reduce bias. The Health Research Authority developed a training module that was informed by the WHO's key criteria, and the group convened in two virtual training meetings to prepare for the review of SARS-CoV-2 CHI models (Davies, 2023). This approach to independent review enabled careful scrutiny of the protocols that were submitted, including the question of whether the CHI models were justifiable after the authorization of highly effective vaccines that protected against severe disease from SARS-CoV-2. Although reasonable people might disagree about the substance of the decision to approve these studies, and other review committees in other countries did not approve SARS-CoV-2 CHI models, the process appears to have been conducted at a high level and with a great deal of transparency.

Engagement with Relevant Parties

Researchers conducting the UK CHI models engaged with members of the public in advance of conducting the CHI models. Pilot research followed by a mixed-methods study involving surveys and focus groups were conducted specifically to assess attitudes and concerns about SARS-CoV-2 CHI models (Barker et al., 2022). While participants generally focused on the potential contribution of these models to speeding up availability of vaccines and treatments, which have not been borne out, one participant mentioned the idea that "We must explore all possible avenues to ensure we find a cure for this miserable virus before it costs more lives, more jobs, more misery" (Barker et al., 2022). It is unclear from the reporting whether this quote reflects a widely shared view or just one person's opinion, however.

Additionally, another fascinating quote from this analysis raises interesting questions about a potential risk that has not been discussed much in the literature: "I think the other risk here is that, if it doesn't produce anything useful or anything beneficial, then you might lose public support . . . or it's not actually speeded anything up. . . . We've been promised all this and then it's not happened, kind of scenario, and that can be as damaging." More research would be valuable to assess whether members of the public perceive that the UK's CHI models offered sufficient value to deliver on prior promises or whether the limited value of the findings to date could actually diminish or damage public support for CHI research.

One concern particular to the development of the UK CHI was that the process was not very transparent or committed to data sharing. The protocol was not published before the process of developing the CHI model began (Morrison, 2021). Additionally, data were published in a preprint more than a year after the study was completed. The researchers who developed the UK CHI models did not share basic information early on to promote the conduct of CHI research by others using similar approaches so the data from different research could be combined.

Lessons for CHI Research with Other Emerging Infectious Diseases

One natural question that arises from examining CHI research with Zika virus and SARS-CoV-2 is whether CHI research can be useful for emerging infectious diseases. Early on in the course of an emerging disease, so much is unknown about how that disease will act in people and what its long-term effects will be. That makes it difficult to evaluate how risky creating a CHI model would be. Yet the possibility of using CHI research for emerging infectious diseases is tantalizing. As some have suggested, "extraordinary diseases require extraordinary solutions" (Plotkin & Caplan, 2020). So, are there circumstances where CHI research for an emerging infectious disease would be clearly ethically justifiable?

One easy case is when CHI research can be done on related strains of a pathogen that we know a lot about and only cause mild illness, particularly if there is an existing model that has a solid safety record. Returning to COVID, conducting CHI studies of cold-inducing coronaviruses would be a smart way to learn more about the disease and ultimately work toward a vaccine that can be used against multiple coronaviruses. This suggestion was made early in the pandemic (Halstead, 2020) because much of what we knew about coronaviruses transmission early on came from the CHI studies conducted by the UK's common cold unit (Tyrrell, 1992).

Influenza is another example where CHI research might be more justifiable with strains that emerge as serious threats to the global population. Some strains of influenza have pandemic potential and may also be likely to be most serious in people with immune systems that do not work very well (i.e., children, older people, and immunocompromised people). Conducting CHI research with young, healthy adults using a strain of influenza that is known to be most serious for those who are immunocompromised could build on the knowledge that has been accumulated over many years about influenza and might be a justifiable way to conduct a CHI model with a pathogen that is causing a global pandemic.

Of course, other pathogens could cause a global pandemic. The WHO has listed several infectious diseases as high priorities for future pandemic preparedness, such as Nipah virus, Ebola virus disease, Rift Valley fever, and Lassa fever. All of the diseases the WHO has prioritized, however, have high mortality rates that would make it very difficult to justify deliberately exposing participants to them to develop a CHI model (Palacios & Shah, 2019). Indeed, as noted in Chapter 3, the highly influential ethical guidelines issued by the Council for International Organizations of the Medical Sciences explicitly call out only two examples of any type of research that exceeds the upper limit of allowable risk. The examples they cite involve CHI research with Ebola virus diseases and anthrax, given their high mortality and the limited treatment options (Council for International Organizations of Medical Sciences, 2016). It is difficult to imagine an ethically acceptable study involving deliberate infection of participants with a disease that has a high risk of death and no good intervention to mitigate that risk. Although it may be possible to use attenuated strains of these pathogens, or related viruses, another challenge is that many of these families of pathogens can cause serious, long-term harm even short of death. As just one example, Rift Valley fever is one of the diseases being monitored for its pandemic potential because it can cause high fever and uncontrolled bleeding that leads to death. There is an uncomplicated form of Rift Valley fever that has a milder presentation, but even that can lead to blindness or long-term neurological complications in the longer term (Anywaine et al., 2022). There is also a concern, even if the probability is low, that such research could lead to a pandemic if sufficient precautions were not taken.[2]

With Ricardo Palacios, I have examined some important conditions for conducting CHI research with an emerging infectious disease and tried to imagine whether there are any examples of conducting such a CHI that would not be ethically controversial. In addition to standard ethical criteria for conducting research, we outlined the following conditions for a CHI with an emerging infectious disease: (1) there is a group that has capacity for consent and is highly likely to have no severe symptoms or death from the disease, (2) researchers could take steps to ensure the disease would not spread to third parties, and (3) the research could be conducted in a place where there was a high background rate of infection (Palacios & Shah, 2019). Notably, while these three conditions were arguably met by COVID-19 CHI models, other conditions matter, too—such as the uncertainty of long-term risks for participants and the value of conducting the research—which rendered COVID-19 CHI research controversial. Before developing a new CHI model to address a pathogen causing a pandemic, the burden of justification will generally need to be high.

The example Dr. Palacios and I used was of a CHI with an emerging infectious disease that we called Disease X that could be relatively easy to justify ethically. This disease would be extremely severe in children

---

[2] I thank Zeb Jamrozik and Katherine Littler for putting on a WHO workshop to address the use of CHI research for pandemic preparedness that helped me develop my thinking in this area.

but only likely to cause mild illness in adults. We imagined a disease that was an enterovirus (an RNA virus that infects people via the gastrointestinal tract) transmitted by fecal–oral or oral–oral contamination and that could also cause brain damage in young children whose neurological development was still ongoing, with a high mortality rate. This type of virus would be relatively easy to contain in a CHI model, and the most serious consequences of the disease would be unlikely to manifest for adults. We imagined this enterovirus was declared a Public Health Emergency of International Concern and several vaccine candidates had been developed. To rapidly select which vaccine candidate to prioritize for future testing, we proposed the development of a CHI model with this pathogen (Palacios & Shah, 2019).

Yet, with the experience of developing COVID vaccines in mind, if Disease X was rapidly spreading, it is not clear that creating a CHI model would be the most efficient way to accelerate vaccine testing. We, however, imagined that a broad coalition of stakeholders agreed on the creation of the model and wanted to use it in various ways. If multiple possible uses of the model could be identified in advance, and if these stakeholders were committed to using it, it is possible to imagine a scenario in which the risks for a CHI model with Disease X were low and the potential benefits were substantial.

Another possibility is that infection challenge models could be developed in nonhuman animals, such as primates. There is a history of intentionally infecting rhesus macaques with Ebola and cynomolgus macaques with Marburg virus (Barnhill et al., 2016). While research with great apes and chimpanzees in particular have been deemed ethically problematic and eliminated in most, if not all, cases, there are still other nonhuman primates or other animals who could be involved in controlled infection studies. In many of these studies, it is important to recognize that the risks would be very high. The exposure of nonhuman primates to diseases that have pandemic potential in humans would likely involve serious risks; one study of Marburg virus has a greater than 40% fatality rate among nonhuman primates simply as a result of infection (Glaze et al., 2015). Moreover, many such studies end with the sacrifice of the animal in order to learn more about how the pathogen has affected different parts of the body. Anne Barnhill and colleagues have argued that "harmful primate research is justifiable only when it is integral to a research program that offers substantial benefits, in terms of the human mortality or morbidity averted, over all ethically permitted alternatives" (Barnhill et al., 2016). They argue for a presumption against doing infection challenge studies with nonhuman primates, particularly if these studies involve only marginal scientific yield. Alternatives, they point to trials with animals that have less cognitive ability, proceeding directly to field research with humans, and CHI studies that are ethical to conduct. They also call attention to the need for anesthesia or palliative care for animals who are suffering. They set a high bar for when such studies could be justified, including that study interventions could prevent significant harm to many people, the experiment is better than the ethically permissible alternatives for alleviating harm to humans, and the study is able to be translated to humans to impact the larger research program.

Ultimately, it may be that the prospect of using CHI research for emerging infectious diseases blinds us to a more likely and important use for such research. The urgency of and fear-based response to emergencies set up an environment for exercising faulty judgment about whether and when CHI research could be useful. The search for "desperate measures" led to the misguided embrace of a method that many ethicists did not fully understand to solve a problem it was ill-suited to address. Rather than focusing on infecting people with pathogens about which we know very little, a better approach might be to expose people to pathogens that we know a lot about but lack the resources to address.

Conclusion

CHI research was touted as a silver bullet solution when it seemed like vaccines would be the key to ending the COVID-19 pandemic. Now we know better and have seen that CHI research in the COVID-19 pandemic did not live up to the hype in the face of a rapidly evolving virus (Hou et al., 2022), vaccines developed at record speed that offered high protection against disease (Kyei-Barffour et al., 2021), and vaccine hesitancy (Omer et al., 2021). We also know that CHI research has important limitations, takes time to set up; this means that if governments are willing to put their money on the line, accelerated vaccine trials can move much more quickly than CHI research. While some have suggested making CHI research faster by skipping the key step of isolating the virus with which people would be infected, the scientific rigor with which CHI research is now conducted is not worth sacrificing in the heat of an emergency (London & Kimmelman, 2020). As we saw in Chapter 1, historical research that involved shoddy science led to confusing results and grave harm to research participants.

The example of Zika virus illustrates that CHI research is a valuable back-up plan for traditional field trials when a pathogen recedes without going away. CHI research may also be important as a component of pandemic preparedness to help build understanding of pathogens well in advance of a global health emergency. For example, CHI models and CHI studies using different strains and related viruses could help to build up a body of knowledge about coronaviruses that might help improve our defenses against them—a move that seems prudent in light of the millions of people who have been harmed or killed by SARS-1, Middle East respiratory syndrome (MERS), and now SARS-CoV-2.

Ultimately, however, focusing on emerging infectious diseases may be a distraction from the most important use of CHI research. There are many pathogens that continually infect people in lower- and middle-income countries (LMICs) and for which there are limited resources to develop interventions. For these pathogens, which may not be newly emerging but still cause substantial suffering and death, the use of CHI research to accelerate the development of vaccines and treatments may be invaluable. We next consider the recent expansion of CHI research to include people in LMICs, along with the potential use of CHI research in so-called vulnerable populations.

6

CHI Research with Newer Populations

When I read about the history of previous Human Challenge Trials [HCT], the successful implementation of an HCT for Typhoid in Zimbabwe caught my attention. I was born in Zimbabwe and grew up there. My childhood was privileged yet I did observe the terrors of diseases in underprivileged communities, especially those affected by HIV. I left Zimbabwe when I was 19 years old, came to America for higher education, and was fortunate to remain and work to get US Citizenship. In seeing that Zimbabweans had risen to an HCT challenge for typhoid that I could do something to address the global crisis of COVID-19 by volunteering for its HCT.

—Prospective volunteer for COVID-19 CHI research

In the past, many of the most ethically troubling cases of controlled human infection (CHI) research involved groups that are sometimes referred to as "vulnerable"—children, people who are incarcerated, unsuspecting patients, and people who live in low- and middle-income countries (LMICs). With the advent of greater regulation and scrutiny of research in the late 1970s, CHI research with these groups largely came to a halt, in keeping with Carol Levine's observation that "the ethical conduct of research . . .was born in scandal and reared in protectionism" (Levine, 1988).

Yet recent developments have called into question whether the exclusion of "vulnerable" groups from CHI research was the right response to historical injustice. Some have pointed out that "vulnerability" is applied loosely enough that almost anyone could fall into that category (Denny & Grady, 2007). Samia Hurst has argued instead that

Intentionally Infecting Humans. Seema K. Shah, Oxford University Press. © Seema K. Shah 2026.
DOI: 10.1093/9780197667927.003.0006

vulnerability should refer to those at heightened risk of being harmed or wronged, with specific attention to the ways in which they could be wronged or harmed guiding how to develop appropriate protections (Hurst, 2008). Members of the Second Wave initiative took aim at the exclusion of pregnant people from research, arguing that pregnant people should not be considered vulnerable at all because there is no reason pregnant people could not give their own consent to research and protect their interests and those of their fetuses. Rather than protecting pregnant people *from* research, this influential group has argued it is better to protect pregnant people *through* responsible research (Lyerly et al., 2021). Ethical guidelines and regulations have taken note and removed pregnant people from those considered "vulnerable" (Council for International Organizations of Medical Sciences, 2016; Office for Human Research Protection, 2018).

These theoretical advances are making their way into the practice of CHI research. Some have recently questioned whether children should be excluded from CHI research (Binik, 2024; Murphy et al., 2020), and a research group recently published what seems to be the first CHI protocol for pregnant people (Theodosiou et al., 2022). Additionally, there has also been tremendous growth of CHI research in LMICs. This research has helped address the limitations of CHI models developed in high-income countries (HICs) that did not generalize to the target populations in LMICs and to make progress against diseases that have long suffered from research neglect (Jamrozik & Selgelid, 2020a).

This chapter aims to clarify when it is appropriate for CHI research to expand into different populations. It builds on the framework presented in Chapter 4 and argues that the categorical exclusion of any group from all CHI research is difficult to justify in general. While it is generally a good idea to exclude those who are truly vulnerable (e.g., unable to consent for themselves) from a novel CHI model, CHI studies can take a more inclusive approach. In CHI studies, it makes more sense to have a default of excluding people at increased risk of harm from a particular pathogen and then consider whether there are special reasons to include particular populations that may be at higher risk. If so, extra protections may be necessary before those populations can be enrolled. Perhaps one reason that the default approach has been to exclude groups considered vulnerable is that there has been limited recognition of the fact that CHI research falls along a wide spectrum of risk.

With that in mind, I first examine recent advances in the concept of vulnerability in the ethics literature. I then explore the recent expansion of CHI research into LMICs and address associated ethical controversies. For example, many CHI studies in LMICs include unusual inclusion/exclusion criteria, such as limiting participation to medical students or people who are interested in participating for altruistic reasons. Additionally, the increased attention to decolonization in research conducted in LMICs has not been applied to consider whether and when CHI research in LMICs is ethically appropriate (Abimbola & Pai, 2020).

Next, I consider whether children should be excluded from CHI research. There are ways CHI research could be designed to fall within the range of permissible risk–benefit ratios for research with children to make it possible to approve under existing regulations (Office for Human Research Protection, 2018). I then consider whether CHI research with children can be not only legally permissible, but also ethically appropriate. Finally, I address whether CHI research should be permitted in pregnant people. Ultimately, I argue that the most important issue in deciding whether CHI research should be open to different groups is considering the risk–benefit ratio and that, for CHI studies that pose low net risk or offer net benefit, a more inclusive approach to recruitment will be easier to justify.

While I argue that the categorical exclusion of any group from all CHI research is difficult to justify, it remains important to learn from historical examples of CHI research with populations that have been called "vulnerable" to ensure that the inclusion of newer populations is not done in a way that echoes past abuses or threatens public trust. I also consider how the distinction between models and studies should map on to CHI research with newer populations. Recall that, in Chapter 4, I argued that the creation of a new CHI model is more ethically complex than the use of an established model in a CHI study. Here, I apply this insight to argue that a similar distinction should be made between developing a new CHI model and adapting an established CHI model to a new population that may be at heightened (or different) risk. CHI models should not be created for the first time in populations at heightened risk and/or that are unable to give their own consent and protect their interests.

Vulnerability in CHI Research

Ethicists have generally argued that "vulnerable" groups should simply be excluded from CHI research, and participation should be restricted to healthy adults who have the capacity to make their own decisions. For example, Miller and Grady reasoned as follows: "In view of the level of discomfort and lack of benefit posed by infection-inducing challenge experiments, this type of research should not be conducted with groups of subjects particularly vulnerable to exploitation. Accordingly, children and incompetent adults, as well as prisoners, should not be recruited for these studies" (Miller & Grady, 2001). Others have included even stronger language that also rules out participation in CHI research for pregnant people: "It is implicit, but perhaps should be stated explicitly: groups traditionally seen as vulnerable in research, such as children and those unable to give informed consent, should be systematically excluded from experimental infections. Corollary to this, it should go without saying that pregnant and lactating women should also be systematically excluded" (Metzger et al., 2019).

As a practical matter, excluding any member of a group that has been considered vulnerable could make it difficult to enroll anyone in CHI research. There is a long list of people who have been considered vulnerable for the purposes of deciding who should enroll in research, including not only children, prisoners, incompetent adults, and pregnant people, but also people with lower incomes or educational levels and racial and ethnic minorities (Denny & Grady, 2007). In fact, in their seminal paper on the ethics of CHI research, Miller and Grady expressly advised against excluding people with lower incomes. They argued that concerns about exploitation could be addressed with a robust informed consent process to ensure that those enrolled were fully informed about the risks involved (Miller & Grady, 2001). Grady later argued that people who are economically disadvantaged should be included in research more generally and that both the informed consent process and external review is important to ensure that research is not taking unfair advantage of participants by offering them a bad deal (Denny & Grady, 2007). Holly Lynch and colleagues have developed a reasoned framework for payment in CHI research that does not require exclusion of lower-income people and further argues that paying participants too little could raise concerns of exploitation (Lynch et al., 2021).

With regard to vulnerability more generally, Samia Hurst and colleagues have forcefully argued that, rather than painting with a broad brush when identifying vulnerability, it is more effective to consider specific vulnerabilities that lead to a heightened risk of being harmed or wronged (Tavaglione et al., 2015). Hurst characterizes this as a shift toward "tailored protections for different forms of vulnerability, rather than blanket protections that may be ineffective or even counterproductive" (Hurst, 2014). Authors of ethics guidance documents have taken note. The latest version of the World Medical Association's Declaration of Helsinki has updated its guidance on vulnerability to focus investigators' attention on specific vulnerabilities that participants may have and ways to address them (World Medical Association, 2013).

In this chapter, I take my cues from this shift in research ethics and focus on specific types of vulnerabilities—examining whether CHI research should exclude people from LMICs, children, and pregnant people. I argue that categorical exclusion of these groups from all CHI research is hard to justify while highlighting specific protections or complexities that may need to be addressed to conduct research with these groups ethically, including making a general distinction between their enrollment in CHI models and engagement in CHI studies.

LMICs

For many years, there has been a perception that conducting CHI research in LMICs raised significant ethical concerns (Jamrozik & Selgelid, 2020a). This may have been based on historical examples of unethical research. The US government conducted CHI research on sexually transmitted infections in Guatemala that was so egregiously wrong it was deemed "ethically impossible" (Presidential Commission for the Study of Bioethical Issues, 2011). It is therefore unsurprising that there has been some wariness about expanding CHI research into LMICs in the modern era.

In 2017, a meeting of the International Alliance for Biological Standardization on CHI research directly addressed the question of whether it was acceptable to conduct CHI research in LMICs. In a publication reporting the meeting results, the authors highlighted that "An important outcome was the proposal that vulnerable populations suffering a heavy disease burden might be considered for inclusion in CHIs that significantly advance vaccine development, particularly when other populations cannot provide adequate surrogate data" (Baay et al., 2019). More recently, Zeb Jamrozik and Michael Selgelid's analysis of the ethical considerations involved in conducting CHI research in LMICs went much farther than merely considering people in LMICs for inclusion. These authors noted that some commentators argue in favor of an "ethical imperative" to conduct CHI research in LMICs (Jamrozik & Selgelid, 2020a) based on the idea that CHI research can help advance treatments and vaccines for infectious diseases that cause high disease burdens in LMICs, such as neglected diseases.

Neglected diseases are those that primarily affect people in LMICs. The World Health Organization (WHO) has identified 20 neglected tropical diseases of high priority. Some are well-known diseases that have long plagued humans, such as leprosy/Hansen's disease and Dengue fever. Others are more obscure, such as yaws, onchocerciasis, and schistosomiasis. While diseases like leprosy are close to being eradicated, Dengue fever infected more than 100 million people and was responsible for the deaths of 40,000 people in 2016 (World Health Organization, 2020). These neglected diseases identified by WHO are not priority problems for wealthier countries, and progress against them is held back by long-standing underinvestment in research. To the extent that CHI research can accelerate work on particular diseases at a relatively low cost (Roestenberg et al., 2018), it holds great potential for addressing diseases that have historically been neglected.

Interest in conducting CHI research also comes from the recognition that data collected in LMICs will have increased relevance for people living there. For example, data from CHI research in HICs on diseases that were not endemic did not translate well to the populations for whom interventions were being designed. CHI research with malaria led to the development of experimental vaccines that were very effective in people who had never been exposed to malaria before and much less effective in people who had multiple exposures to malaria throughout their lifetimes. This led to the realization that controlled human malaria infection models needed to be developed with people who had been exposed to the disease to advance a successful malaria vaccine (de Jong et al., 2021)—most of whom could be found in LMICs.

In light of the increased interest in expanding CHI research in LMICs, the Wellcome Trust led an effort to build capacity to conduct CHI research in LMICs and commissioned two ethicists to address ethical issues related to CHI research in endemic settings (Jamrozik & Selgelid, 2020b). Given the name of this project, it is worth briefly explaining the difference between research in endemic settings and research in LMICs.

In the early days of the expansion of CHI research, a common view was that CHI research in HICs was being conducted on naïve populations where particular infectious diseases were not circulating rather than in endemic settings where many people had prior exposure to the disease, and moving the research to LMICs was necessary to remedy that. However, this terminology was somewhat misleading because whether a disease is endemic in a setting is different from whether that setting is a HIC or an LMIC. In fact, many CHI studies have been conducted on diseases that are endemic in high=income countries, such as adenoviruses that cause colds and influenza, and SARS-CoV-2 in the United Kingdom. The real shift was that there was greater interest in conducting these studies in LMICs instead of in HICs, which requires investment into capacity-building. CHI research is now being conducted in some LMICs (e.g., Kenya, Zambia, and Vietnam) on diseases like malaria and dengue (Hodgson et al., 2014; Kestelyn et al., 2019; Shekalaghe et al., 2014). Countries like India that have not previously permitted CHI research are also considering investing in this research method for the first time (Sharma et al., 2022). Despite the potentially confusing terminology, Jamrozik and Selgelid's report was ultimately published as a book that provides a helpful entrée into CHI research in LMICs.

Ethical Considerations for CHI Research in LMICs

Jamrozik and Selgelid identified five major ethical considerations for CHI research in endemic settings—or, as noted above, in LMICs: (1) informed consent, (2) undue inducement, (3) transmission of infection to third parties, (4) capacity to review ethically complex research, and (5) public perception of these studies. Drawing on their work, I review each of these in turn. First, however, I note that the distinction between models and studies is as relevant here as it is elsewhere. The initiation of CHI research in a LMIC for the first time adds extra complexity, such as the need to build capacity in conducting research and overseeing it or considerations about how to prevent third-party risk. Accordingly, the development of a new CHI model is not how an LMIC—or, really, any country—should begin conducting CHI research.

Returning to the criteria laid out by Jamrozik and Selgelid, the first one relates to informed consent. Obtaining valid informed consent in CHI research has often been assumed to be more difficult in LMICs than in HICs. Scholars have raised concerns that participants from LMICs may have additional difficulty understanding the concept of deliberate infection and the level of risk involved because of language barriers, low literacy, and/or low health literacy (Vaswani et al., 2020). Accordingly, some CHI research conducted in Vietnam, Kenya, and Tanzania requires participants to be students or to have a certain level of educational attainment, such as a secondary school certificate (Hodgson et al., 2014; Jongo et al., 2018; Kestelyn et al., 2019). As noted in Chapter 4, exclusion of people based on their perceived ability to understand is not required for ethical reasons. In a co-authored paper with Vina Vaswani and colleagues, we argued that exclusion of people from LMICs based on assumptions about their ability to understand violated the principle of fair participant selection. The assumption of more limited capacity for understanding in LMICs could also be faulty. Indeed, participants from LMICs where a disease is endemic might have a greater understanding of what it means to be deliberately infected with that disease than participants from HICs who have never seen anyone who had the disease (Vaswani et al., 2020).

Taking an evidence-based approach to address concerns about informed consent is also important. Reassuringly, data on comprehension of research do not demonstrate substantial differences between people from HICs versus LMICs (Mandava et al., 2012). There are some aspects of research that are hard for people to understand no matter where they live, such as randomization or placebo use. Some studies suggest, however, that people from LMICs may have more difficulty understanding that they are free to withdraw from research at any time.

Given that CHI research can include restrictions on withdrawal to protect third parties outside of the research from being infected with the pathogen (Fernandez Lynch, 2020), this is an important issue that should be addressed with data-driven approaches to informed consent. And as noted in Chapter 4, the data on informed consent suggest that the most effective ways to ensure understanding are relatively low tech, such as test–feedback approaches (Flory & Emanuel, 2004). Tests of understanding seem to be widely used in CHI research and could emphasize that participants can withdraw from research at any time but may put themselves or others at risk if they leave isolation while infectious. In addition, they may not be able to come out of isolation if they are infectious, depending on local laws (Vaswani et al., 2020).

There are also ways to improve understanding of informed consent that are culturally specific. For instance, some CHI researchers found through community engagement that presenting the amount of blood that would be drawn during the study in spoons rather than milliliters would be easier for participants to understand. Others have described randomization using examples related to farming—specifically, creating illustrations of farmers planting seeds in two different ways in two different fields to see where the yield is greater (Ndebele et al., 2012). Thus, using data-driven approaches to informed consent is a reasonable way to address concerns about enrolling people living in LMICs into CHI research without being unnecessarily paternalistic by simply excluding these populations.

Second, Jamrozik and Selgelid argued that concerns about undue inducement can also be raised if participants are likely to be paid larger amounts of money for their participation in CHI research in LMICs than they might be able to earn outside of the research. Determining what counts as fair compensation for research participation can be especially challenging in LMICs. Neal Dickert and Christine Grady developed a wage-payment model for determining how to pay research participants fairly. This model focuses on the kind of work that is asked of participants and then determines what is fair to pay them based on the economic market. In the United States, the model suggests that the low skill level required of research participants merits minimum wage (Dickert & Grady, 1999). However, in some LMICs, there is no set minimum wage (Center, 2021). There can also be wide variation within a country or minimal enforcement of minimum wage laws to ensure that people are compensated fairly. This places extra burden on ethics review committees and institutions in LMICs to develop practices and policies around payment that can ensure participants are compensated appropriately for the time and burdens involved with research.

Third, concerns about transmission to third parties may arise in LMICs if there is a vector that can transmit the disease outside of the research setting. Importantly, this issue is not specific to LMICs—consider CHI research with SARS-CoV-2, influenza, or adenovirus in countries like the United States or the United Kingdom. Any of these viruses could be transmitted by participants to research staff or to others if they withdrew from the study early, and some diseases can also be transmitted by vectors like mosquitoes or through water and sewage systems. Capacity to do these studies in a rigorous and safe manner (given the need for insectary facilities to house the mosquitoes and to conduct parasite cultures) was a key consideration when CHI malaria research moved from being conducted in HICs (where there were no mosquitoes that could transmit malaria in the surrounding area) to LMICs that had mosquito species that could transmit malaria (Sheehy et al., 2013; Shekalaghe et al., 2014). Additionally, CHI research with enteroviruses that are transmitted through contact with bodily fluids might pose a higher risk of third-party infections in countries where the sewage system and infrastructure is less developed. However, with strong capacity-building efforts, CHI studies with malaria have now been safely conducted in LMICs, some of which infected participants through injection of parasites (Jongo et al., 2018; Shekalaghe et al., 2014). This suggests that concerns about third-party risks are important and require attention, but can be overcome.

Jamrozik and Selgelid's fourth consideration for CHI research in LMICs is that it should be reviewed by independent committees that have sufficient capacity to review it and under a regulatory scheme that provides guidance for the most salient ethical considerations. In the past, some countries lacked clear systems of regulation for CHI research. Several steps have been taken in recent years to build capacity, from developing international guidance for the review of CHI research to countries like India and Kenya developing their own internal guidance specific to CHI research, as discussed further below. It is important to recognize that review committees can have different kinds of blind spots that are not limited to LMICs. For instance, a review committee in the Netherlands faced with a protocol for a schistosomiasis CHI may have experience in reviewing CHI research but lack experience related to the disease, while the reverse may be true for a review committee in Uganda. Thus, the need to build capacity is not necessarily an HIC–LMIC distinction but may be important to address in LMICs regardless.

Finally, community perceptions of CHI research in LMICs are important to consider and may be colored by historical abuses. Some communities may fear that CHI research is being done in LMICs rather than HICs because it is risky and that the benefits and burdens of the research will not be shared fairly (Vaz et al., 2021). Perhaps more fundamentally, with increasing attention to the importance of decolonization efforts in LMICs, there is also a concern that CHI research might exacerbate rather than ameliorate long-standing injustices. This concern merits further examination.

Use of CHI Research in LMICs and Decolonization Efforts

Underinvestment in neglected diseases is not simply due to the small numbers of people who are affected by them; rather, it stems from the legacy of colonization and attitudes of supremacy. Local forms of knowledge were often suppressed or damaged by colonizers, to be replaced with paradigms that were more familiar to them. Research agendas were set primarily based on the needs of colonial powers; overlap with the needs of local people typically was limited to situations when colonizers felt the impact of a disease on their workforce. In the modern day, investment in diseases continues to track with how much of a priority a disease is for higher-income countries (Packard, 2016). Research agendas are often defined by and largely funded by HIC governments or international organizations that are run by and based in HICs, inevitably leading to less research on diseases that primarily occur in lower-income countries (Packard, 2018). Scholars have argued that even the term "global health" has a legacy of oppression and injustice and that if "global health" were to truly be decolonized, it might be so unrecognizable that it should be called by another name entirely (Abimbola & Pai, 2020).

Whether CHI research can serve to help fill unmet research needs of LMICs without undermining decolonization efforts is an important question. First, if CHI research is led and driven by people and priorities from HICs, it may fail to address the needs of people from LMICs and could reify existing injustices. Yet there may be ways to address this concern. For example, attending to mechanisms for sharing power and incorporating meaningful community input may help improve accountability and relevance to people in LMICs (Pratt, 2021). From a more pragmatic standpoint, there are times when the interests of HICs and LMICs may align, and these opportunities may be worthwhile for LMICs.[1] For instance, with increasing awareness of the pandemic potential of diseases that are currently seen mostly in LMICs, there has been interest in developing vaccines for neglected diseases like Nipah virus (Khan et al., 2024).

Additionally, as described in Chapter 1, there is a historical legacy of unethical international CHI research, including CHI research with sexually transmitted infections conducted by the US government in Guatemala and research conducted by the Nazis that led to

---

[1] I would like to thank Vivian David Jacob for highlighting the potential alignment between HIC and LMIC interests.

the development of the Nuremberg Code (Presidential Commission for the Study of Bioethical Issues, 2011). That legacy may make it difficult for various publics to trust the introduction of new CHI research into LMICs and suggests that research about public attitudes, education, and country-specific guidance for CHI research may be needed as researchers seek to expand into LMICs.

Third, the uncertainty and risk associated with some CHI research, particularly with neglected diseases, may raise concerns about exploitation of participants. Importantly, some neglected diseases are treatable, which makes it easier to justify conducting a CHI with these diseases because the risks are low. While CHI research has been conducted successfully in some lower-income countries, such as Kenya and Thailand, ethical concerns about CHI research in India has held back its use, with recent guidelines from the Indian Council of Medical Research (ICMR) being an important milestone in moving this research forward, as discussed further below. The lack of trust in the Indian government in the context of recent research ethics scandals may make it difficult for people to embrace the concept of using CHI research to address local health problems (Vaz et al., 2021).

Finally, it is also possible that the rationale for doing CHI research on neglected diseases merely adds insult to injury. One of the key reasons to consider CHI research is that it can also provide large returns on small investments of time and effort, which could be of great value for underfunded diseases. Yet to say to people in LMICs that underinvestment in solving their problems is likely to persist—unless they are willing to agree to conduct riskier and cheaper studies where participants are deliberately infected with diseases—may not be a message that is well-received, and for good reason (Hughes, 2012).

One key question is to what extent LMICs see CHI research as ethically concerning and what problems they think are important to address. The development of country-specific guidance can be an important way to ensure that contextual considerations are taken into account. The first country-specific guidance about CHI research was developed in Kenya, in September 2022, although these guidelines were embedded within general guidelines about research. In 2023, the ICMR issued a policy statement to support the ethical conduct of CHI research in India. Ethical issues highlighted in this policy include concerns about "ethics dumping" and the exploitation of low-income people who might participate in CHI research for financial reasons (Indian Council of Medical Research, 2023b). Both the process of developing India's policy statement and the guidelines ultimately adopted are instructive for understanding how LMICs that have been wary of CHI research for ethical reasons might begin to allow CHI research to be conducted ethically within their borders. Below, I review these two guidance documents for insights into how CHI research can be expanded into LMICs with ethical and cultural considerations in mind.

Kenya's Guidelines for the Conduct of Clinical Trials

In 2022, the Kenyan Ministry of Health included CHI research in its guidance for the conduct of clinical trials. This guidance focuses on "Controlled Human Infection Studies" and generally does not distinguish between models and studies except in one key place. Section 1.453 says that "CHI model models should be developed in maximally resourced settings before introduction to Kenya." This suggests that the guidelines contemplate the use of CHI studies in Kenya and not the creation of new models. When defining these studies, the guidance notes that they are "trials in which participants are intentionally challenged with a well-characterized pathogen in a controlled manner while being closely monitored" (Republic of Kenya Ministry of Health, 2022). Thus, the studies are framed as careful from the outset, perhaps with the goal of reassuring the public that it is reasonable to permit them.

The guidelines focus on ensuring that the potential benefits justify the risks, and rely on the importance of the disease burden in Kenya as the way to determine whether a study has sufficient social value. There is also an appreciation of the potential risks to third parties and the need to prevent infection for study staff and others outside of the study. There are several provisions related to limits on risk and the need to minimize risk. For example, the guidelines contain a great deal of information about strain selection, including testing the strain used to infect people to ensure it is free of other pathogens, and using the lowest potency of the strain needed to reach the scientific endpoints.

The guidelines explain that the strain used should "ideally" be manufactured in accordance with Good Manufacturing Practices (GMPs)—a high standard of quality control that is not required in all countries, including the United Kingdom. Another way that risk is minimized is through the requirements that "robust" clinical care be provided to participants and insurance for research injury is purchased. Finally, the Kenyan guidelines set an upper limit of risk of sorts by stating that it would not be appropriate to do CHI research if there was a high chance of fatality from the disease, there is a long and uncertain period before infection emerges, or if there are no therapies for the disease that "preclude death."

Notably, some of the language in Kenya's guidelines appears to focus on the concern of double standards—that LMICs should not host research that would not be ethically acceptable elsewhere. Ruth Macklin has raised this concern with respect to the use of placebo controls in research (Macklin, 2021), and these guidelines seem designed to address worries that CHI research conducted in LMICs might raise the same ethical issue. The language requiring CHI models to be developed in "maximally resourced countries" is a key example of this, along with language stating that the clinical facilities must ensure that the risk is not greater than if the study was conducted in another part of the world.

Within the guidelines, there is no section specifically focused who should be enrolled in these studies, but people at increased risk of complications from the disease are to be excluded. The guidelines also specifically mention that they are focused on research with adults and that pregnant people should not be included unless there is a "compelling rationale and justification." Thus, children are implicitly excluded and pregnant people are subject to a default of exclusion unless there is a good reason to include them. There is no mention of exclusion on the basis of education or health literacy. Instead, the guidelines sensibly focus on the need to conduct robust informed consent that also informs participants that, even if they withdraw from the study, they may have to remain under quarantine. It is also considered ideal that participants take a test of understanding before enrolling.

One final protection is that boards to monitor data and safety (referred to as Data and Safety Monitoring Boards or Data Monitoring

Committees) are recommended for all CHI studies. This is not standard practice for CHI research but could be a useful way of maintaining oversight by a group of experts appointed by the study sponsor who would review data from the study while it is ongoing and could recommend whether to stop, modify, or continue the research.

Country-Specific Guidelines

The ICMR released a draft policy statement for public comment in July 2023 and held an "Indo-U.S. Workshop on Clinical Research Ethics and Challenging Newer Areas" that included discussion of this draft on August 7–9, 2023. After soliciting peer review and public comment, the ICMR published a final version, in December 2023, that incorporated responses to the feedback received (Indian Council of Medical Research, 2023b). The motivation for this guidance was to carefully consider whether and how to start permitting CHI research. As one participant stated in the August 2023 workshop, "Research was a bad word in India, and has evolved to be a neutral word in the COVID pandemic. Should we wait for it to be an excellent word [before allowing CHI research]?"[2]

Unlike other guidance documents, the ICMR policy statement does distinguish between CHI models and CHI studies, albeit to a limited extent. For instance, the policy statement tackles the question of whether and how to start CHI research in India. The policy statement first explains the difference between CHI models and CHI studies and then states that the first CHI research in India should involve the use of an established CHI model with a strong track record of safety to minimize both the ethical complexity of the research and the risk of losing public trust.[3]

Elsewhere, the document largely drops the distinction between CHI models and CHI studies. The terminology used throughout the policy statement refers to CHI studies only. Although this may be a semantic issue to some degree, there are also substantive omissions.

---

[2]   Author's notes from workshop attendance on August 7, 2023.
[3]   This author was consulted on the language referenced in this paragraph.

For example, the document does not consider whether a novel CHI model should be reviewed more stringently than the use of an established model in a CHI study.

The ICMR policy statement was influenced by the WHO guidance reviewed in Chapter 4 but departs from it in ways that are both negative and positive. In what follows, I focus on examining those differences. First, the positive. The ICMR instructs review committees to focus on researcher competence in and experience with ICMR guidance. A focus on researcher competence and experience may be particularly important in India given that CHI research has not yet been conducted there and researchers may bring training from other sites to build capacity to do CHI research. It may also be important for review committees to consider researcher competence and experience for the development of a new CHI model anywhere. (Poomkudy & Shah, 2024)

Another virtue of the ICMR guidance is its ability to draw on existing guidelines in India for compensation for research-related injury. In stark contrast to the United States, India has extensive regulation for compensation for research-related injury (Larkin, 2015). The United States only requires that participants are told whether or not they will be compensated if they are harmed (and it is legally acceptable not to provide any compensation for people who are injured by their participation in research) (Henry et al., 2015). This section of the ICMR guidance adds to existing guidelines by noting the possibility that insurance could also be purchased for third parties outside of the research, depending on "the nature of the infective organism or where the risk is higher" (Indian Council of Medical Research, 2023b).

With respect to other differences between the ICMR's guidance and WHO guidance, they may reflect concerns particularly important for India and other LMICs. However, the approaches that are recommended to address these concerns may add to existing confusion. For example, the policy statement raises and attempts to address concerns related to "ethics dumping" but does not provide much clarity on what this term encompasses. At the Indo–US Workshop in August 2023, this issue was hotly debated. Participants were unable to coalesce around a specific definition of "ethics dumping" but generally felt that it occurs when research is sponsored by higher-income countries and does not address the health needs of LMICs. This view of "ethics dumping" seems similar to the concept of "responsiveness" in research (Council for International Organizations of Medical Sciences, 2016; World Medical Association, 2013). To address this concern, the policy statement requires that any CHI research done in India should address diseases that are "prevalent in the country" presumably because of the sense that it is necessary to ensure that the benefits of research accrue to people in India. However, as has been noted in debates about responsiveness, there can be reasons for conducting research to build capacity that may not directly map on to current health problems in the country but that could be important for accelerating higher-priority research in the future (Shah et al., 2013). Furthermore, one strategy to prepare for future pandemics would be to conduct CHI research on strains that are related to pathogens that could cause pandemics, such as CHI models with coronaviruses that only cause mild cold-like symptoms in healthy people. By including the requirement of disease prevalence to prevent ethics dumping, this policy might unintentionally limit the ability of Indian researchers to build capacity and advance pandemic preparedness.

Similarly, another issue raised in the ICMR policy statement that may foster confusion was motivated by concern about the exploitation of vulnerable populations in India. The document defines "vulnerable" participants as "are those who have limited autonomy and are either relatively or absolutely incapable of safeguarding their own interests due to personal disability, environmental burdens, social injustice, a lack of power, understanding, or the ability to communicate or they may find themselves in situations that prevent them from doing so" (Indian Council of Medical Research, 2023b). While the first part of the definition focuses more narrowly on capacity to consent, the idea of "situational" vulnerability could have much broader applicability. As noted earlier in this chapter, the field of bioethics is moving away from such a broad definition of vulnerability because of the recognition that if most people are vulnerable, this may lead to overprotection and default exclusion (Hurst, 2008). Over time, overprotection in research limits the generalizability and access to the benefits of research for many groups (Tavaglione et al., 2015).

To address vulnerability, the policy statement focuses on one particular type of vulnerability—people with low education levels—and requires that CHI participants should be graduates from a college or a university (at least). However, as noted in Chapter 4 in the discussion of informed consent, it is not clear that higher education is necessary or sufficient to help ensure participant understanding. Use of evidence-based methods to ensure understanding of the research can help to address barriers faced by people from various educational backgrounds, and education does not necessarily predict the ability to understand what it means to be in a study involving deliberate infection with a particular disease. Some participants who may not have a great deal of education may have more knowledge and experience related to a particular disease if they have seen others become infected with it in their community (Vaswani et al., 2020).

Notably, the first draft of the policy statement was more restrictive about who could participate in CHI research. The document initially required that researchers enroll participants who were altruistic and should withhold information about the amount of payment until *after* the participant had given consent (Indian Council of Medical Research, 2023a). This requirement was removed in the final version, which now acknowledges that there is no good way to determine whether a participant is engaging in research for purely altruistic reasons. Many studies have demonstrated that participants typically have mixed motivations, hoping to advance science and earn money in the process (Stunkel & Grady, 2011). Additionally, any participant who was motivated by money could always withdraw from the research after finding out how much they were being paid. Although these difficult-to-enforce approaches to ensuring altruism are no longer in the ICMR policy statement, the final policy still expresses discomfort with the possibility that some people might participate in CHI research for monetary motivations.

Finally, unlike WHO guidance documents, the ICMR policy statement includes a section on post-study access, benefit sharing, and publication. This section requires researchers to communicate with review committees and participants about intellectual property arrangements in advance of and after the study and to share benefits if there are any. While benefit-sharing has received increased attention, with some ethicists arguing that it may be ethically advisable to distribute the benefits of research fairly, how to share benefits in practice remains unclear (Johnson & Wendler, 2015). If a product is developed after several studies have been conducted (including studies with negative results), many research participants might have a claim to the benefits of the research. Even from a purely logistical perspective, compensating all participants for such claims would be challenging. Sorting out how much should be owed to different participants based on factors like the level of risk they undertook and the phase of research they participated in would raise difficult normative issues that have not been resolved.

Examples of Efforts to Conduct Ethical CHI Research in LMICs

In recent years, there have been a few examples of CHI research being introduced in other countries in an ethically sensitive manner. Efforts to develop a schistosomiasis CHI to be used in Uganda and to introduce CHI research in Kenya may be particularly instructive in providing a path forward that is attuned to the needs of people in LMICs.

For readers unfamiliar with schistosomiasis, some background may be helpful. Schistosomiasis is a parasitic infectious disease that causes serious harm and death around the world but primarily in several countries in Africa. *Schistoma* worms live in blood vessels around the human bladder or gut. Female worms lay eggs that are excreted in stool or urine. The eggs hatch in water and then enter a snail that serves as an intermediate host that then sheds larvae, which reenter humans through bathing, swimming, or other exposures to water containing the larvae. While most infections are asymptomatic, the symptoms can include delayed fever and infection, and more serious complications can occur due to the body's reaction to the parasite's eggs, which can spread to other tissues, including the brain. When the eggs enter the human liver, they can cause progressive liver fibrosis, portal hypertension, and even death through uncontrolled hemorrhage (Nelwan, 2019).

There are no authorized or approved vaccines for schistosomiasis. The main intervention for this disease is a treatment called praziquantel, which is widely administered in endemic settings. Although some countries, like Uganda, have used the strategy of mass drug administration, this has proved insufficient to eradicate the disease. People who are cured of schistosomiasis can be infected again, and drug resistance could develop. Developing vaccines is challenging because these parasites have evolved to evade the human immune system. Weakened organisms have induced immunity in some animals, but producing these organisms at scale is not feasible, so vaccines are being developed using antigens from the organisms. Vaccines using these antigens are at various stages of development, but because there are limited resources to address this disease, vaccine development moves slowly. Animal models are also not ideal for studying schistosomiasis (Koopman et al., 2021). There is clear potential social value from the development of a CHI model with schistosomiasis in light of these challenges and what a CHI model could contribute. First, a CHI model could help identify a correlate of protection, which could speed up the process of testing vaccines and treatments by serving as a surrogate marker. A CHI model could also be used to select the best of existing vaccine candidates or to test new treatments.

To advance a CHI model for schistosomiasis, a research team first developed the model in the Netherlands at Leiden University Medical Center, an institution with a great deal of experience in conducting CHI research. In the CHI model, several steps were taken to minimize risks. To avoid the morbidity caused by the eggs of the parasite, the first model infected participants with only male larvae, and a follow-up model used female larvae, given important biological differences between the immune response based on the sex of the larvae and the greater resistance of female larvae to existing treatments. The CHI model required following participants for 12 weeks until they were cured of infection through successful treatment. The snails and larvae were manufactured in facilities dedicated to this work and followed GMP principles (Koopman et al., 2023).

The research team recognized, however, that developing a model in a place where schistosomiasis is endemic could help determine how prior exposure to the parasite affects the efficacy of different vaccines.

Importantly, they worked to determine whether developing a CHI model was ethically acceptable and aligned with local priorities *before* moving the model to Uganda. The research team convened stakeholders in Uganda to discuss the ethical and scientific issues surrounding the creation of this model (Egesa et al., 2022). Stakeholders raised a number of issues, including the need to develop a full community engagement plan that involved key opinion leaders. Although other CHI research in LMICs focused on recruiting medical students, people attending the meeting in Uganda felt that students are still dependent on their parents and that their parents might object to their participation in a CHI. Interestingly, this concern is somewhat universal because qualitative studies in the United States have found that participants have faced opposition from their parents, with some mothers offering to pay participants the same incentive they would get from trial participation if they did *not* participate in CHI research (Kraft et al., 2019).

This engagement also revealed a positive reason to do CHI research in LMICs. One participant who worked with communities living on island communities in Lake Victoria that are heavily affected by schistosomiasis strongly supported the conduct of schistosomiasis CHI research in Uganda. He said that a vaccine was urgently needed and that communities would see the urgency, be capable of understanding the risks involved, and be willing to participate. This underscores the fact that communities that live with particular diseases are likely to understand the risk of deliberate infection with that disease better than communities that have limited, if any, experience with those diseases (Egesa et al., 2022).

As another example of robust community engagement before introducing CHI research into a new country, Dorcas Kamuya, Melissa Kapulu, and colleagues engaged with communities in Kilifi, Kenya, before and during the conduct of CHI studies with malaria (Mumba et al., 2022). They convened a large community advisory body of approximately 200 representatives that the researchers could consult with to share information, find out what the perceptions of the research were, and consider how the study should be designed.

This approach had several benefits. For instance, engagement with the community representatives led to the quick identification of unsubstantiated rumors that were circulating about the study and the ability to address them quickly. Additionally, community engagement helped disseminate information about the study early to improve the quality of informed consent that was later obtained from volunteers. Regular interactions between the study team and community members also helped to demonstrate respect and build trust. Interestingly, one challenge that the team faced was that their engagement with members of the media appeared to backfire when an article was published in the newspaper about the study that made it sound as though the study was paying people large amounts of money for taking on high risk. However, the main response to the article was that many people contacted the study team because they were interested in participating—a surprisingly positive response that the team had not anticipated. Ultimately, the team was able to respond to the article with a press statement that was posted to social media (Njue et al., 2018). These examples demonstrate how CHI research can be done in LMICs to a high ethical standard and may help support the conduct of increasing amounts of CHI research in LMICs in the future.

Children

The prospect of conducting CHI research in children raises considerable unease for many people. As discussed in Chapter 1, historical examples of CHI research with children would be considered ethically problematic in the modern era and unlikely to be approved by an ethics review board today (Davies, 2007). Recall that Edward Jenner inoculated his gardener's 8-year-old son, James Phipps, with cowpox, thinking that this would protect him against subsequent infection with smallpox. Jenner then exposed Phipps to smallpox more than 20 times to test whether cowpox infection would protect him (Ellis, 2021). This research was ground-breaking in that it proved the concept of vaccination. Yet the risks of his approach were highly uncertain, and it could have been lethal to expose Phipps to smallpox. A modern-day defense of Jenner has been mounted by bioethicist Hugh Davies (Davies, 2007). Davies has defended Jenner by arguing that the risks of cowpox exposure were lower than the fatality from variolation, which was a common practice at the time. Yet Jenner's approach raised other ethical concerns aside from the risk. It is unclear how much information was shared with Phipps and his family in advance or whether they gave permission.

The Willowbrook hepatitis challenge studies, also discussed at greater length in Chapter 1, are perhaps the most prominent and debated example of CHI research with children. These studies raised a great deal of controversy, particularly over their use of institutionalized children. Indeed, the first ethical debate on CHI research came directly from the conduct of these studies when Henry Beecher called them out as unethical (Beecher, 1966), and the investigator leading these studies, Saul Krugman, publicly defended the ethics of his work (Krugman, 1971, 1986). There have been other, lesser-known examples of CHI research with children involving diseases like typhus and trachoma. Typhus is a disease that is spread by lice, which has a high rate of mortality in adults and a much lower case fatality rate in children. In the 1930s, researchers conducted studies in Tunis in both adults and children were inoculated against typhus with small doses of infectious material, presumably justified by the fact that children were at much lower risk from inoculation than adults. However, the details of these studies are scant, and the few publications on them are in French. It is unclear what, if any, ethical protections accompanied the enrollment of children in this CHI research (Murphy et al., 2020).

In the 1960s, three children with blindness who were between the ages of 12 and 14 were enrolled in challenge studies involving trachoma (Bernkopf et al., 1964). Trachoma is a bacterial infection that, without treatment, can lead to blindness. Other symptoms include itching and irritation of the eyes and eyelids, discharge of the eyes, swelling of the eyelids, light sensitivity, pain, and redness (Potter, 1993). The researchers noted that they asked the children questions about any symptoms they were experiencing several times, and found that "subjective symptoms were practically absent" (Bernkopf et al., 1964). Researchers did notice some objective symptoms that they meticulously documented, including thick, greenish secretions in the infected eye; atypical thickening of the eye membranes in two of the three children; and swelling of the lymph nodes. The researchers provided treatment to the children once the "clinical picture had become sufficiently definite," which was less than 40 days after exposure to the bacteria. Notably, the researchers addressed concerns about spread of the infection to the child's other eye and considered the risk of infecting third parties by closing the infected eye with a perforated metal sheet. It is difficult to evaluate the ethics of this research with the information available, but there are open questions about whether the study could have been conducted in adults with the capacity to consent.

Given the troubling history of the inclusion of children in CHI research without sufficient ethical protection, it is no surprise that the early ethics literature on CHI research recommended the exclusion of children altogether. Yet recent publications have cast some doubt on the practice of categorical exclusion. For instance, Jamrozik and Selgelid conducted interviews with 45 experts on the ethics of CHI research and found considerable controversy on this question. They ultimately described "widespread consensus" that "even if disease-causing [CHIs] in children could be conducted safely, there should be a presumption against enrolling children in such studies" (Jamrozik & Selgelid, 2020b). These experts favored alternatives to CHI research on children when possible, such as conducting CHI research with adults or field trials in children. If CHI research was to be conducted in children, they argued that the following requirements should be met: (1) a strong scientific rationale, (2) international consultation, and (3) community engagement demonstrating acceptance.

The United Kingdom's Academy of Medical Sciences also convened a workshop in which the issue of enrolling children and pregnant people in CHI research was debated. Some participants worried that the exclusion of children and pregnant people from CHI research could result in the denial of access to beneficial interventions for these groups. They advocated for considering inclusion while exercising "extreme caution" to address concerns about public trust, but did not elaborate further (Academy of Medical Sciences, 2005). In a subsequent meeting by the same organization in 2018, participants raised similar concerns about it being discriminatory to exclude children and pregnant people from CHI research. Yet the meeting participants ultimately concluded that "CHI model studies which involved such vulnerable groups should be considered with extreme caution as there is both a high ethical risk and a risk of loss of confidence in research ethics if an approach was ill-advised" (Academy of Medical Sciences, 2018).

WHO guidance also suggests that it may be ethically acceptable to include children in CHI research. The general guidance document for all CHI research notes that,

> Paediatric CHI study may be permissible where they comply with research ethics standards that characterize the additional protections required when enrolling participants who may lack appropriate decision-making capacity. These include restrictions on acceptable risk and burden profiles, and requirements for assent (in keeping with the child's capacity) and parental or guardian permission (World Health Organization, 2022).

Later in the document, the WHO adds that prior relevant research should be conducted in adults and that public engagement is critical for such research because it has the potential to damage public trust.

In collaboration with two CHI researchers and a social scientist, I have examined whether the categorical exclusion of children from CHI research is justifiable (Murphy et al., 2020). In our paper, we argue that children have been excluded from CHI research based largely on the assumption that all CHI research poses relatively high risk. If this assumption were correct, CHI research with children would not be legally permissible as international regulations only permit children to be enrolled in research that has low net risk or a potential for benefit that outweighs the risk (Wendler & Varma, 2006). This regulatory framework is based on ethical concerns that children do not have the capacity to consent and protect their own interests.

In our paper, we demonstrate that the assumption that most CHI research poses high risk is inaccurate. Rather, CHI research falls on a spectrum from very low to very high risk, with some studies possibly offering potential for benefit. In particular, very-low-risk studies include CHI studies that use live attenuated vaccines as the challenge strain. Indeed, CHI studies with licensed, live-attenuated pathogens have been conducted in children (including some infant studies) with intranasal influenza virus vaccine (Belshe & Van Voris, 1984), rotavirus vaccine (Groome et al., 2017), and polio vaccine (Brickley et al.,

2018). These CHI studies used vaccines that were already approved for use in children as the challenge strain to test new vaccines. For example, children were given a new inactivated poliovirus vaccine and then challenged with the oral, live-attenuated polio vaccine to provide robust data on whether the new vaccine worked, which was tested by determining whether children shed poliovirus afterward.

As we noted in the article, one might respond that these types of studies should not be considered CHI research. To this way of thinking, using a live attenuated vaccine is not the same as using a challenge strain that has been developed specifically for the purpose of doing a CHI study (Murphy et al., 2020). While it is true that the approach of using a licensed, live attenuated vaccine is generally a safer one than developing and testing a new strain, this is a difference in the *degree* of risk, not the nature of it. Moreover, as we note in the paper, dengue CHI studies are clearly considered CHI studies even though they use a strain that is a live attenuated vaccine that was never approved.

Even assuming for the sake of argument that studies using live, attenuated vaccines as the challenge strain should be distinguished from other CHI research, there are other types of research that inarguably count as CHI studies and are low net risk. For example, CHI malaria studies have a long track record of safety and are a routine part of the process to develop new interventions for malaria. In standard CHI malaria studies, participants are infected by mosquito bite or injection with a strain of malaria that is not resistant to treatment (Stanisic et al., 2018). After someone is exposed to malaria, malaria parasites move through an initial stage before making it to the bloodstream to cause illness. Malaria parasites first develop in the liver without causing any detectable symptoms. After 5 or 6 days, they enter the blood and multiply rapidly, causing illness 10–15 days after they were transmitted by mosquito. Once malaria can be detected in the blood with a standard assay, participants in a standard CHI with malaria will receive treatment and be cured, with no lasting effects.

Although CHI malaria studies have enrolled thousands of volunteers without serious side effects, they could be done in a manner that is even lower risk. If CHI malaria studies were to involve children, CHI studies with malaria could be done by giving participants the treatment medication *at the same time* that they are exposed to the challenge strain, thus ensuring participants are protected from the start. Given the length of time it takes for malaria parasites to make it from the liver into the bloodstream, in the lower-risk study imagined here, participants would be cured before experiencing any symptoms. Furthermore, when the approach of challenging people who already have treatment on board is done repeatedly with a relatively high dose of challenge parasites, it has been shown to confer protection against future malaria infection (Bastiaens et al., 2016), suggesting that participants may have a chance of benefit that could at least partially offset the risk.

This hypothetical example suggests that there could be a way of designing CHI research that involves low net risk and could be approvable under existing regulations. Of course, many other research procedures pose risks that would have to be considered to determine the balance of risk and benefit, including blood draws and time spent in a research facility. While these procedures add some degree of risk, they also decrease the risk of serious complications from infection. We assume here that the risks of these procedures do not increase the risk substantially.

Clearly, there are examples of high-risk CHI research that would not be easy to justify in children, such as CHI research with influenza (Roestenberg et al., 2018). Higher-risk CHI studies are ethically problematic to conduct in children because they lack the authority to authorize their own exposure to risk. Parents also lack moral and legal authority to expose their children to high risk of harm. These ethical concerns are reflected in the regulatory structure that governs pediatric research, and higher risk CHI research would not be legally permissible under existing regulations.

Once we dispatch with the argument that all CHI research is too risky to include children, however, several other ethical issues remain that may still pose challenges for including children in low-risk CHI research. We have argued that several other ethical issues should be addressed, namely: (1) there should be compelling scientific justification for enrolling children (including that there are no alternative approaches to learning similar information), (2) the study should provide compensation for research-related injury, (3) the study should involve robust community engagement and should not be done if there are strong views in the community against the inclusion of children in CHI research, (4) robust approaches to informed consent and assent should be followed (if appropriate), and (5) researchers should not force any children to participate in research even when they lack the capacity to assent and are not asked for their acquiescence prior to enrollment (Murphy et al., 2020).

One challenge with these conditions is that it is not straightforward to ensure a child is not being forced to participate in research under existing regulations. Informed consent processes for studies involving children typically include asking for parental permission and child assent, to the extent the child is capable of giving their assent. Even for children who are not capable of understanding what research involves, however, it can be important to respect their expressions of distress or dissent (Bos et al., 2017). A child who experiences severe distress at research participation is being subjected to additional harm beyond what was contemplated when the research was approved, harm that could increase the risk of the study to an unacceptable level. Additionally, if a child refuses to undergo research procedures, research staff may not be willing to restrain the child to complete the procedures. The act of being restrained may also cause psychological harm to a child. Thus, the informed consent process should be designed to ensure that children are engaged to the extent they are capable, and children who are likely to change their minds about research participation should not be enrolled. If a child dissents from research, they should be allowed to withdraw from the research itself as soon as possible and be able to leave the research facility as soon as it is safe to do so.

Another issue that relates to the growing autonomy of children is which group of children to enroll. In general, we also felt it important that CHI research use *age de-escalation* (Murphy et al., 2020), which simply refers to the idea that older children should be enrolled prior to enrolling younger children, in recognition of the fact that older children have more developed autonomy and can participate more in decision-making about the research.

Finally, other issues we were unable to fully resolve related to confinement and payment. If a study required confinement to protect participants or third parties, it would be problematic to require young children to be confined apart from their parents. If their parents were confined with them, however, this would likely require enrolling the parents in the study as it might be difficult to prevent them from becoming infected. Involvement in such a study could prove burdensome, particularly for parents with more than one child. If parents were asked to take on the burden of confinement, they should also be provided with compensation for their time, which could end up being substantial.

Compensating parents for their child's participation in CHI research could raise several thorny issues. Payment for pediatric research is a contentious issue that has received limited attention. The standard view on payment for research with children is that it is important that payments will benefit the child directly, to recognize the fact that they are the ones who participated in the research. However, given the level of commitment required for CHI research, it would make sense to compensate parents for the time and burdens they undertake to ensure their children are able to participate. Higher amounts of payment, including for the participation of parents, could then increase the possibility that parents would enroll their children in research for the money and potentially coerce their children to enroll and remain in the study against their will. For these reasons, we concluded that CHI research requiring confinement of children would likely be ethically problematic (Murphy et al., 2020).

A more recent ethical analysis of CHI research with children similarly came to the conclusion that it could be ethically acceptable under a limited set of conditions (Binik, 2024). Binik did not address the issue of payment in her article and was less concerned about confinement in CHI research, suggesting that more research is needed on the views of parents and children about confinement and whether there are ways for it to be acceptable to them.

Binik had three main disagreements from our analysis of the enrollment of children that are worth examining further, specifically arguing that (1) there should be a scientific necessity requirement for including children in CHI research, (2) there should be a presumption against the inclusion of children in CHI research, and (3) age de-escalation should be approached in a nuanced way. First, Binik argued that it was not sufficient to require a compelling scientific justification for enrolling children, and researchers should be required to demonstrate that it is scientifically necessary to include children in CHI research. Notably, when the National Commission for the Protection of Human Subjects was first considering whether to permit pediatric research in the United States, there was a heated debate over whether children should be allowed to participate in research that was not beneficial to them. The arguments that won the day concluded that children should not be enrolled in nonbeneficial research unless it was scientifically necessary to include them rather than adults, although this was not clearly reflected in the regulations that were ultimately developed. It is not entirely clear how the scientific necessity requirement dropped out, but ultimately, the US federal regulations imposed a requirement that if more than minimal net risk research with children is permitted, it should only be done if there is a chance it will benefit the condition that the participants suffer from (Shah & Wendler, 2010). For CHI research, Binik may be right to draw on this concept of scientific necessity to ensure that children are only enrolled when necessary. A further modification of the requirement may be needed, however—the scientific question being asked should have sufficient social value to justify the risk. If it is only possible to answer a question that is not that important by enrolling children (assuming of course that the study was important enough to justify the risks), it still may not be justifiable to conduct CHI research with children.

Second, Binik argues in favor of a presumption against CHI research with children, which could be reasonable but requires further specification. It is not clear how strong of a presumption Binik has in mind and what level of evidence would be needed to overcome it. Such a presumption may go too far if it makes it impossible to conduct low-risk or net-benefit CHI studies that might involve children, particularly CHI studies with live attenuated vaccines that pose very low risk, if any.

Third, Binik argues that although age de-escalation seems advisable for CHI research for scientific and other reasons, age de-escalation may need to be approached in a nuanced way (Harbin et al., 2023). In particular, while autonomy is one important consideration, another factor that can be more important is the level of risk. If younger children are at lower risk than older children for some reason, this may be a reason to conduct CHI research with younger children, which is a point well-taken.

One limitation of both Binik's article and the previous piece we published on CHI research with children is that they do not consider the ethical relevance of the distinction between models and studies. It seems clear that children should generally not be included in novel CHI models that lack any experience in adults. Even if a novel model was being established that was determined to pose low net risk, which is difficult but not impossible to imagine, it would still be important to have experience with the model and data establishing its safety in adults. In other words, to be a candidate for the inclusion of children in CHI research, the CHI model would have to first have an established track record of safety in adults unless there was some reason this was not possible and the model was thought to be low risk with evidence coming from another source (such as models that use licensed live attenuated vaccines).

Thus, while this analysis reveals that some of the discomfort at the thought of CHI research involving children may be based on a misconception that all CHI research is high risk, there are still many other reasons to be cautious about conducting CHI research in children. The categorical exclusion of children from CHI research is not justifiable, but several protections should be in place for such research to be conducted. Now that we have tackled the controversial issue of involving children in CHI research directly, there is also one other type of CHI research that could indirectly involve children that would benefit from further examination for its own sake—specifically, CHI research with pregnant people.

Pregnant People

There has long been a dearth of research with pregnant people (Lyerly et al., 2008). An ethos of extreme caution toward research with pregnancy grew out of the tragic consequences of the use of drugs that turned out to cause severe birth defects, such as thalidomide to treat morning sickness and diethylstilbestrol (DES) to prevent complications from pregnancy. Yet pregnant people continue to have health needs, both related and unrelated to their temporary state of being pregnant. The near-complete exclusion of pregnant people from research for many years has had serious consequences. For example, the failure to include pregnant people in early vaccine trials in the COVID-19 pandemic led to confusing guidance about whether pregnant people should be vaccinated, lower uptake of the COVID vaccines among pregnant people when they were available, and, ultimately, increased mortality among pregnant people from COVID-19 (Whitehead & Walker, 2020).

In light of this history, scholars founded the Second Wave Initiative, a collaboration between academics and others to develop evidence for the treatment of pregnant people. As part of this work, Annie Lyerly and colleagues have argued for three conceptual shifts regarding the inclusion of pregnant people in research. First, they have proposed reclassifying pregnant people as "complex" instead of "vulnerable." Second, they advocate for protecting pregnant people *through* research rather than *from* research. Third, they argue for a shift from a default of presumptive exclusion to an approach involving fair inclusion (Lyerly et al., 2021).

Lyerly and colleagues explain that pregnant people should not be classified as "vulnerable" because the protections developed for so-called vulnerable populations are not necessarily relevant for them. In contrast to children and adults with limited cognitive capacity, pregnant people have the capacity to consent. And, unlike people who are incarcerated, pregnant people are not necessarily more likely to be exploited or coerced. These important insights have been incorporated into ethical guidelines and regulations. For example, both the WHO's Council for International Organizations for the Medical Sciences and the US Department of Health and Human Services have indicated that pregnant people should no longer be considered "vulnerable" (Council for International Organizations of Medical Sciences, 2016; Office for Human Research Protection, 2018).

Yet the reevaluation of research with pregnant people has not yet spilled over into the literature on the ethics of CHI research, with few authors addressing the inclusion of pregnant people unless they are explaining why pregnant people should not be enrolled in these studies (Durbin & Whitehead, 2017; Jamrozik & Selgelid, 2020b;

Metzger et al., 2019). There is good reason for caution because some infectious diseases can be worse in pregnancy or cause harm to infants, such as COVID-19 and Zika virus. Thus, without thinking through their inclusion in CHI research, research could cause considerable harm to pregnant people and fetuses without corresponding benefit. Nevertheless, the reflexive exclusion of pregnant people from research has harmed pregnant people as a group and is an injustice that should be corrected.

With respect to whether to include pregnant people in CHI research, it makes sense to consider the case of research that is important to conduct in pregnant people and poses low net risk, because such research could be permissible under existing regulations. For example, US federal regulations require that research offers a prospect of benefit for the pregnant person or fetus, or, if not, less than minimal risk is posed to the fetus and the research is being done to produce important knowledge that cannot be obtained otherwise (Office for Human Research Protection, 2018).

As an example of what acceptable CHI research in pregnancy might look like, researchers have published what appears to be the first protocol that outlines an approach to CHI research in pregnancy. Unsurprisingly, this research involves low risk and a prospect of direct benefit to pregnant people and infants (Theodosiou et al., 2022). This CHI model involves inoculating people late in pregnancy with *Neisseria lactamica*, a bacteria that is not harmful and can be beneficial. It is well known that infants acquire beneficial bacteria from their mothers, and the goal of this study is to test whether inoculation of the pregnant person can ultimately contribute to the microbiomes of the infant and protect them against upper respiratory tract infections like meningitis. In adults, CHI with *N. lactamica* was associated with a 10% decrease in the bacteria that causes meningococcal disease (e.g., meningitis and bloodstream infections). Although there is a vaccine that protects against meningitis, this vaccine is not designed to be taken in the first 2 months of life, and infants are at high risk of having invasive disease if they are infected at that time.

The *N. lactamica* CHI model for use in pregnancy therefore seeks to build on the prior development of a CHI model in which 400 adults who were not pregnant were exposed to this bacterium by the same research group, and it was found to be safe and reliable (Dale et al., 2022). The researchers planned to enroll two groups: (1) participants who already have colonization in the nostril with the bacteria and (2) those who do not, who will undergo CHI. The idea behind including the first group is that the researchers can do an opportunistic study looking at whether pregnant people who have the bacteria already pass it on to their infants. Notably, prior to conducting the study, the researchers did a qualitative study to assess the attitudes of pregnant people toward participation and found general interest along with concerns about risks (Dorey et al., 2023). In light of their findings from the qualitative interviews, the research team minimized the risk of the study further, including by omitting a previously planned blood draw in newborns (Theodosiou et al., 2022). While there might be ways the study could be ethically improved, for example by exploring alternatives, the key point here is to recognize that this type of research suggests an example of CHI research with pregnant people that is ethically defensible.

It is also important to recognize that concerns about the inclusion of pregnant people in CHI research may have had unintended consequences. In particular, worries about including pregnant people have led to the widespread exclusion of people from CHI research who identify as women when they are of reproductive age, which is even more concerning. It is not uncommon for CHI studies to only enroll males (Dabira et al., 2023). In one CHI study with malaria, a participant who was a transgender female was initially told she was not eligible to participate, but the researchers reconsidered when she explained that their concerns about pregnancy would not apply to her (Kraft et al., 2019). More data are needed about the gender breakdown of participants in CHI research to determine the significance of this problem (Adams-Phipps et al., 2022). Yet it would not be surprising if concerns about pregnancy during CHI research may cast a long enough shadow to lead to the exclusion of women of reproductive age. Such exclusion limits the generalizability of this research in ways that may not be at all necessary, provided participants are willing and able to remain on effective and reliable contraception throughout the study. As we saw in the discussion of a Zika virus CHI model in Chapter 5, there may even be some instances in which it is safer to enroll women in CHI research to minimize risks to third parties outside of the study.

Objections

This chapter has generally argued against categorical exclusions of groups that were traditionally considered vulnerable, suggesting that any categorical exclusion of a group from all CHI research would be hard to justify. Some might balk at the idea of dismantling categorical exclusions of groups from all CHI research, arguing that because CHI research raises an unusual set of complex and/or unresolved ethical issues, surely there is some category of people who should not participate in CHI research for their own protection. For example, many people have the intuition that only "healthy" people should be engaged in such research. This seems reasonable to minimize risk in many cases, and people who are healthy prior to their enrollment in CHI research could be assumed to be at lower risk than others. Additionally, if people are not infected with other diseases, scientists can better control the circumstances of infection, which is important for CHI research.

Even this attempt at identifying a category of people who should be excluded from CHI research fails, however. CHI studies with malaria have been conducted with people living with HIV whose condition was well-controlled on antiretroviral therapy (Jongo et al., 2018). This was done to ensure that malaria vaccines could be tested in people living with HIV who make up a significant proportion of the population in some countries where malaria is endemic. Admittedly, given the safety of CHI studies with the established malaria model, the notion of developing a model to test vaccines in people living with HIV is easier to justify than enrolling participants in other models might be. Additionally, people living with HIV who are well-controlled on antiretroviral therapy are healthy, for almost all intents and purposes. If CHI studies become more widely used as a part of the process to test new vaccines and treatments for many diseases, CHI models that have been shown to be safe in healthy people might become commonly tested in people living with HIV or other conditions in the future.

As another example of a categorical exclusion that appears justifiable but may not be, during the COVID pandemic, there was widespread agreement that only young, healthy people should be enrolled in CHI research (Eyal et al., 2020; Jamrozik et al., 2021), and researchers recruited participants in line with this view (Killingley et al., 2022). Some argued to the contrary, suggesting that CHI models would be able to more accurately assess whether vaccines and treatments worked in the people at highest risk from COVID-19 if older people were enrolled (Matsui et al., 2021). Strikingly, in a study we conducted examining the motivations of volunteers for CHI research to address COVID-19, we found that 111 people who volunteered (5.8% of those in the study) who were over the age of 65. Twelve people who were 76 or older signed up on the registry (Marsh et al., 2022). This raises the question: Should older people who are willing, able, and eager to participate in CHI research be excluded?

As with any group, perhaps the most critical question is about the risk of harm from participation. To begin with the risk of physical harm, older people tend to have more comorbidities and to be frailer than younger people. Many diseases, like COVID and certain forms of influenza, are much more serious in older than younger people. This suggests that, for many types of CHI research, it may make sense to exclude older people. Yet some diseases are more dangerous for young adults, as was observed during the 1918 influenza pandemic (Gagnon et al., 2013). This suggests that there is the possibility that older adults could be at lower risk than younger adults in some cases.

Furthermore, Matsui and colleagues have argued that, for older adults, "death for them would represent a loss of fewer years of life than it would for the group of younger adults" (Matsui et al., 2021). If harm is defined as setting back one's interests (Feinberg, 1984), then the harm of death can be thought of as lower for older people who have already had many years of life to enjoy and who might have fewer projects left to complete in their lives. Older people who have lived long lives may feel they have less to lose and therefore be willing to take on greater risks for the benefit of others. As a 53-year-old volunteer said: "I am slightly older than most and have had a good life; time to pay it back a little." Another person who identified as female and was 73 years old said, "I think it's better for me, as an older person, to take a risk, rather than someone younger that still has a full life ahead of them." This person recognized she was at high risk but volunteered regardless.

Additionally, some people felt that they should volunteer for CHI research *because* they were older to help provide data for their group. For instance, a 70-year-old woman who volunteered stated, "I think the study needs to include older, healthy people as well as younger people to truly get an accurate picture of how the vaccine will work." Another person who was 63 years old similarly expressed the following sentiment, "I think the most vulnerable people seem to be older people. As I am at the lower end of 'older,' it seemed to me that I would maybe be a more suitable 'guinea pig' for a vaccine." And a 60-year-old said the following: "being in an older demographic, I wanted to help the study be representative of the population" (Jurden et al., 2024).

It is also possible that, in rare instances, enrolling older people might be ethically preferable to enrolling younger people. The Last Gift study discussed in Chapter 3 is a fascinating example of a study that enrolls people who are terminally ill in research to test HIV cure modalities and be able to perform invasive procedures immediately after death to learn more about the viral reservoirs where HIV typically hides inside the body (Riggs et al., 2022). This is a study that takes seriously the idea that people who are coming to the ends of their lives have little to lose and may find meaning in contributing to something larger than themselves. If there was a type of CHI research that had very high risk that was justified by the potential social value, and it could be performed on people who were terminally ill, it might be much easier to justify such a study than to perform it on someone younger and healthier who had many years of life left to live.

In sum, these examples suggest that categorical prohibitions on participation might be reasonable defaults or presumptions (Binik, 2024), but not more than that. The diversity of potential research designs and corresponding levels of risk in CHI research, coupled with the many reasons people might want to participate, can generate ethically justifiable examples of CHI research with populations previously thought to be off the table for recruitment. Perhaps a more accurate way of understanding who should be approached for participation in CHI research is to focus not on categories of people who are widely considered "vulnerable," but to begin with understanding the scientific reasons for doing a particular type of CHI research, identifying the groups that resemble the target population for future interventions against the pathogen, and evaluating and minimizing the risks posed by the research to different groups.

Conclusion

CHI research with so-called vulnerable populations was initially considered ethically impermissible. Recent developments have called into question such a broad and blunt approach to vulnerability. Additionally, the idea that all CHI research poses the same level of risk and that it is always high risk has led to unnecessarily restrictive interpretations of who should be included in CHI research. In this chapter, I have taken the position that CHI research in LMICs can be done ethically and that, although certain issues may merit additional attention in LMICs, they are not necessarily LMIC-specific issues. The only possible exceptions are the need to ensure participants understand their right to withdraw from research and the need to consider the role of a CHI in ongoing efforts at decolonization of health research. Furthermore, I have argued against the categorical exclusion of any group from all CHI research by attempting to demonstrate that groups traditionally considered vulnerable might be able to be enrolled in CHI research ethically, including children and perhaps even pregnant people. As research ethics has moved away from protectionism and toward responsible inclusion, it is time for CHI research to follow suit.

7

How Can the Ethics of CHI Research Help Advance Research Ethics?

Q: Which of these risks and burdens [of a CHI with SARS-CoV-2] concerned you the most?
A: If something goes wrong, it may undermine the public trust in the vaccine and science in general. If people find the trial unethical, it may further enhance reluctance to get vaccinated with this particular vaccine(s) or vaccines in general. The need to find someone who would care for my cat when I'm in hospital/research facility.
—Interview of a volunteer for 1Day Sooner

This analysis of controlled human infection (CHI) research presents an opportunity to consider some broader theoretical and practical implications that extend beyond this unusual type of research, some of which may be surprising or illuminating. Because CHI research presents a central question of research ethics—When is it acceptable to expose some people to risk for the benefit of others?—in stark relief and also raises several complex and/or unresolved ethical questions, this analysis has implications for research ethics more broadly. Accordingly, I turn to exploring whether insights from analyzing CHI research may be able to help the field of research ethics get unstuck on long-standing, unsettled issues. As I demonstrate below, several existing quandaries in research ethics can be better understood and advanced by the contributions gained from a more systematic evaluation of the ethics of CHI research.

Intentionally Infecting Humans. Seema K. Shah, Oxford University Press. © Seema K. Shah 2026.
DOI: 10.1093/9780197667927.003.0007

What Can This Examination of CHI Research Tell Us About Research Ethics More Generally?

Several lessons can be learned from the ethical examination of CHI research. Perhaps the first lesson is that while bioethics scholars sometimes focus on whether there is anything ethically unique or novel about scientific advances (Hsia, 1999), such a narrow focus can miss an important signal that extra ethical attention is warranted. Just as CHI research raises several complex and/or unresolved ethical issues at once, other types of research may raise challenges that are not entirely novel or unique but still worthy of dedicated attention. While prior ethics work can help when a cluster of challenging but not entirely novel issues arise at once, how these issues interact with each other can be unique and difficult to untangle. Thus, dismissing the need for specialized ethical analysis or frameworks simply because there seems to be nothing entirely novel can miss the forest for the trees.

This analysis of the ethics of CHI research also raises five more concrete implications for research ethics more broadly by helping advance understanding of: (1) the need for greater consideration of a potential "yuck" reaction to research, (2) how (or how not) to evaluate social value, (3) whether it is ethically acceptable to raise the upper limit of risk for research in an emergency, (4) the ethical importance of site selection, (5) the ethical complexity of self-experimentation, and (6) the importance of elevating research participants' status in society.

The "Yuck" Reaction

As discussed in Chapter 2, the so-called yuck reaction, where people intuitively respond to something as yucky and therefore ethically questionable, has received limited attention in research ethics. Yet, as we saw earlier, CHI research is far from the only type of research to raise a "yuck" reaction. Examples include research with brain-dead bodies (Wicclair, 2008), research on xenotransplantation of organs from pigs to humans (Platt & Cascalho, 2022), research with people who are engaged in sexual intercourse (Greenberg et al., 2013), and very rapid autopsy on deceased patients in the Last Gift study (Riggs et al., 2022).

There are at least two reasons greater consideration of the "yuck" reaction may be warranted in other areas of research ethics. First, it is possible that the "yuck" reaction limits the conduct of important and valuable research that causes our intuitions to misfire. Second, concerns about public trust in research sometimes focus on potential negative reactions from the public but neglect the possibility of ethical unease from research teams who must carry out the research.

It is impossible to measure the studies that are never done due to concerns that they could raise ethical challenges and would be unattractive to potential participants, but there is no doubt that such examples exist. Studies that are hard to conduct because of the potential for a negative reaction are easier to identify. Perhaps the best example in this regard is the Last Gift study, in which people who are terminally ill volunteer to receive interventions and then have a rapid autopsy conducted after death to advance HIV cure research (Riggs et al., 2022). The Last Gift study stands out among the examples discussed in Chapter 2 because of its unusual nature and the strong initial negative reaction that people might have to it. Yet closer examination of the ethical issues reveals that the ethical issues raised by this research can be addressed (Kanazawa et al., 2023), suggesting that concern about the study may be an example of a misfiring intuitive reaction. It is possible that studies like these have been avoided because of concern about negative reactions from the public. Accordingly, ethicists may have an important role to play in deciphering what a potential "yuck" reaction means for a given study. Embedding ethicists or social scientists in research that has the potential to raise negative intuitive reactions can help examine the likely public response, develop ways to combat public misperceptions, and strategize how to address ethical issues that may arise in a proactive and thoughtful manner (Shah et al., 2022).

Additionally, while the potential for loss of public trust has been discussed in the ethics literature (Hope & McMillan, 2004; London, 2012), along with ways to address this proactively, the intuitive reaction of people more directly involved in conducting research has received much less attention. For example, when a Zika virus CHI model was being considered, ethical concerns arose not at the sponsor or research review stage, but rather when people at the institution began confronting the reality of being involved in a study in which people would be deliberately infected with Zika virus. The reaction of those people critical to the conduct of research is vital and can derail projects if it not considered. Anecdotally, I have been consulted as an ethicist on studies where research teams had ethical concerns that were not addressed and they deviated from the protocol to meet what they felt were their duties to the participants. Ensuring that potential intuitive reactions that relate to ethical concerns are addressed head-on for those involved in research is important for the success of a given study. It may be that their concerns have validity, as was true initially for Zika virus CHI research (Shah et al., 2018), but also that these concerns could be addressed with sufficient attention to the relevant evidence and ethical issues (Vannice et al., 2019). On the other hand, study staff might have concerns that are misplaced or based on a lack of information. Either way, it is important for study teams to acknowledge that these types of reactions might arise and face them directly, both from an ethical and pragmatic perspective.

Uncertain Social Value

Determining the social value of research when its benefits accrue in the longer term can be challenging. Consider basic science research, which is foundational to scientific progress but can occur years or even decades before it has a demonstrable impact on health. Basic science research could lead to negative findings or could uncover insights that may be incorporated into a wide range of other studies that ultimately produce substantial public health benefits. How should the potential social value of such research be considered? CHI research is a helpful lens into this age-old quandary (Rid & Roestenberg, 2020).

Chapter 4, revealed that there is an important distinction between CHI models and the subsequent studies that are done with a model has after it has an established track record of safety. Evaluating the social value of the creation of a single CHI model in isolation can be an inadequate test of whether this research is valuable enough to pursue because it is also important to consider the insights that will be obtained from creating the model and an attempt to forecast how that model might be useful in the future. We saw that one solution may be to recognize how CHI research fits into other ongoing research and that it should be justified in terms of whether CHI research is a key piece of a larger puzzle.

Some scholars have argued that all clinical trials should be understood in this way—as part of a larger research "portfolio" (London & Kimmelman, 2019). London and Kimmelman contend that there are different points on the testing trajectory that are all in service of the goal of finding an intervention that will improve the care of patients in the future. In the early part of the trajectory, research is focused on exploring hypotheses to determine which avenues are worth pursuing further. Later, studies test promising hypotheses, and still later, studies are required to confirm the effects of the experimental intervention within the practices that are already being used to care for the target population. They point out that what most people think of as "silver bullet" drugs that revolutionize patient care are merely the tip of a research iceberg. As an example, they note that the anticancer drug imatinib involved more than 10 years of testing with more than 37 different clinical trajectories and 128 trials. These authors argue that our current system of research oversight focuses too narrowly on individual trials without considering their place in the larger portfolio.

London and Kimmelman note several implications of this problem, including that Institutional Review Boards (IRBs) and their international equivalents do not scrutinize trials that keep exploring new potential trajectories to maximize the potential profits of pharmaceutical companies rather than societal benefit. Additionally, sponsors make many private decisions about research portfolios that are not transparent, despite having significant ethical implications. Submissions to IRBs rarely provide the context of different trajectories that have been tested to explain the particular contribution of the trial being evaluated. The authors recognize the enormity of the problem they have identified and that it will be difficult to implement many of the solutions they propose. CHI research, however, provides some insights into how research oversight could be reformed to address some of these issues.

First, recall that the United Kingdom's regulatory authority that reviewed proposed CHI models spent time in training on how to evaluate these studies prior to evaluating the actual protocol. They even reviewed a mock protocol to prepare (Davies, 2023). The recognition that CHI research is different from many other types of studies facilitated a training process that enabled the review committee to get up to speed on the research design. Perhaps a more fundamental reform of review processes is needed to ensure training of IRBs to understand how individual research studies fit into a larger picture. Another possibility is that there is a need for greater specialization of review committees in disease areas where there is rapid progress and complex trajectories, just as specialized review might be needed for CHI models, or greater consultation with experts when review committees do not have scientific expertise represented on their panels.

Second, even if it is too much to ask of IRBs to review research portfolios in addition to individual studies, this does not mean that a more careful look at social value is beyond our reach—greater attention to recommendations and decisions made by other groups can help fill in the gap. For example, sponsors like the National Institutes of Health (NIH) are increasingly recognizing the importance of negative social value in their decision-making, hiring ethicists to help in internal review of research and convening special panels to review research of heightened controversy (Shah et al., 2018). Some ethicists have already turned their attention to the duties of regulatory authorities and how they should consider social value and other ethical implications in their work (Lynch & Bateman-House, 2020; Mello et al., 2012). Regulatory agencies that can withhold approval due to ethical concerns have important levers for ensuring the ethical conduct of research when it is undertaken by industry. More work may be needed to adequately address how the US Food and Drug Administration (FDA) evaluates individual studies in light of their place in a larger research program.

Ethical attention to the efforts of Data Monitoring Committees (DMCs) is another critical component of research ethics worthy of greater attention that could also help make more complex judgments about social value. DMCs are independent groups of experts that examine unblinded, interim data as randomized controlled trials are ongoing and operate with the ethical imperative to ensure studies do not continue to randomize participants longer than is needed to produce robust evidence (Ellenberg & DeMets, 2016). DMCs play the important function of addressing the social value of research in a dynamic way (Shah et al., 2021) and are well-suited to this task because they include experts with deep knowledge about the landscape of research related to a particular condition who can make recommendations to stop or modify studies when the risk of proceeding outweighs the benefit to others in society. One challenge is that DMCs typically communicate only with sponsors and research teams and enter into confidentiality agreements. This means they cannot easily raise concerns to others if they believe a particular study is ethically problematic because it fails to fit within a larger research portfolio. Developing ways that DMCs can share their ethical concerns with other oversight bodies when they have ethical concerns about the social value of a given study in light of the broader portfolio is an important area for future research.

Finally, the challenge of forecasting how scientific insights will make contributions in the longer term may, somewhat paradoxically, suggest the benefit of a pragmatic approach to studies that do not ethically require careful calibration of social value. While efforts to improve the rigor in assessing potential future social value are important for studies that pose high risks and require high social value to justify those risks, they may be less critical for research that involves lower risk. Review committees that are already overwhelmed may not need to try to anticipate for every study how a particular scientific advance might translate into value in the future and how likely it is that particular contributions will be realized. As long as review committees can determine that a study uses robust scientific methods to answer a question that might have value in the future and the net risks to participants are relatively low, they may not need to formally assess the magnitude and probability of the potential social value before letting the research move forward and can focus more attention on studies that need more careful oversight of social value.

The Upper Limit of Risk in an Emergency

Whether there is an upper limit of risk in research, and if so, what it would be, is an unresolved issue in research ethics (Paquette & Shah,

2020). As discussed in Chapter 4, existing regulations do not place a clear upper limit on risk in research, and ethical guidelines offer little additional help. International guidance documents from groups like the Council for International Organizations of Medical Sciences (CIOMS) typically shy away from setting a specific upper limit on risk. However, the commentary to the CIOMS guidelines explains that, although there should be an upper limit of risk in research, an exact limit is difficult to specify. Accordingly, the authors of the guidelines turned to challenge studies as examples to help determine what level of risk would intuitively be too high to accept. They argued that a challenge study involving deliberate exposure to Ebola virus disease or anthrax would pose risk that is too high to be ethically acceptable in light of present knowledge about these pathogens and available treatments (Council for International Organizations of Medical Sciences, 2016). CHI research is a clear useful illustration and reminder of why an upper limit of risk in research is important. Research involves societal support and is conducted by researchers and at institutions. There are externalities associated with conducting high-risk research in that, if the risk is realized and someone is harmed, this may threaten public trust and the willingness of others to enroll in research in the future. As discussed in Chapter 1, we are still living with the consequences of decades-old, unethical research studies that cast a long shadow on the research being conducted today.

The question of whether there is an upper limit of risk in research becomes especially pressing in an emergency. Interestingly, even those who have argued for an upper limit of risk in ordinary times have suggested that an emergency might permit doing away with risk limits. Steve Joffe and Frank Miller have noted that dire public health emergencies could allow for higher risk limits for research (Miller & Joffe, 2009). Read in conjunction with the CIOMS guidelines, this might lead some to consider whether CHI research that would otherwise be impermissible might be acceptable in an emergency.

In light of the recent experience of the COVID-19 pandemic, however, I would question whether public health emergencies are helpful or harmful ways to test our intuitions about limits on risk. During the COVID-19 pandemic, public trust was often in short supply while being sorely needed for many parts of the pandemic response

(Kennedy et al., 2022). There were different ways to speed up research, each involving complicated ethical tradeoffs. Ultimately, the decision to take enormous financial risks with research, rather than exposing individual people to extra physical risks, produced vaccines much more quickly than developing a new CHI model would have (Slaoui & Hepburn, 2020). Despite the cautious approach taken by public health authorities, decreased public trust, particularly along racial and partisan lines, led to lower uptake of vaccines and many preventable deaths (Dhanani & Franz, 2022). This suggests that the idea that risky research can be easier to justify in an emergency is far too simplistic for decision-making during a pandemic.

A decision to sacrifice public trust can have significant, measurable consequences. Clearly, there is value to building up trust and understanding of scientific methods in non-emergency times, as was the case in the United Kingdom with CHI research (Barnes et al., 2023). With a baseline of public understanding and trust, greater risks in research may be tolerated by members of various publics. Yet in the midst of an emergency, when trust is at a premium and a foundation of trust is not already in place, taking excessive risks in research or engaging in shortcuts may be dangerous and could threaten other aspects of the pandemic response (Kahn et al., 2020). Accordingly—and contrary to suggestions in the existing bioethics literature— an emergency might not be the time to discard the protection of having an upper limit of allowable risk in research.

The Ethical Importance of Site Selection

A related implication of this analysis is that *where* research is done matters morally, for instance, when considering the potential effects of research on public trust. The issue of site selection has not been explicitly been recognized in general frameworks for research ethics, however (Emanuel et al., 2000). Another lesson learned from this analysis of CHI research is that research can have long-term, uncertain harms that may be difficult to assess or provide compensation for through standard approaches. In the United States, several bioethics commissions have addressed the question of compensation for research-related injury ar.d argued that it is ethically important to do (Pike, 2014). The arguments supporting compensation for research-related injury are straightforward and have been made for decades—if researchers cause harm, participants should not be left to subsidize research participation by paying for treatment or other expenses incurred because they are injured. Compensatory justice requires that the person who caused the harm—the researcher—try to make the person who experienced the harm whole again, insofar as possible. Providing compensation and care for injuries that occur during research can also minimize risks, which is widely recognized as a requirement for ethical research (Pike, 2012).

Yet finding an adequate mechanism for ensuring compensation for research-related injury has proved challenging in many countries. In the United States, there is no national scheme for compensation for research-related injury. In India, regulations that required compensation for research-related injury were initially met with a great deal of skepticism by other countries (Larkin, 2015). These regulations were so controversial that the NIH paused all of its sponsored research in India for a few months after they were passed. Ultimately, the United States and India came to an understanding of how the regulations would operate in practice, and the regulations have now been functioning reasonably well over the past several years. Yet what has been missing from this debate and the proposed solutions is the recognition that harm from research may take years or even decades to manifest—and this is something that examining CHI research highlights (Halpern, 2021). Putting the burden on a research team with short-term funding to conduct research makes it very likely that the obligation will go unfulfilled. With most grants only lasting for 5 years at a time, it is unclear how any research team could set up a system on their own to ensure that research participants receive compensation for harm that occurs years later.

CHI research provides clear examples of cases where the harm from research participation took several years to manifest, and the researchers would have found it difficult to provide compensation. For instance, hepatitis challenge trials in the 1950s and 1960s could have led to liver disease and death decades later (Halpern, 2021). With longer-term harm, there is also more of a chance that intervening factors make the assessment of who is responsible for the harm much more challenging. Consider SARS-CoV-2 CHI research, where participants may have had COVID-19 during the trial and later been infected with subsequent variants. If they experienced long COVID or serious complications from COVID infection, the fact that they had been infected in the trial would likely have contributed to the harm. Should researchers be held fully responsible for compensating someone who needed healthcare over time due to long COVID, particularly if the controlled infection the participant received was only one of several infections they had experienced? An additional complication arising in CHI research is that harms to third parties outside of the research may also require compensation, which is explicitly recognized in the guidance issued by the Indian Council of Medical Research (ICMR) discussed in Chapter 6. Furthermore, for trials that are reviewed, supported, and prioritized by a government sponsor, researchers should not have to bear the burden of providing compensation for research-related injury on their own, and the government also bears some responsibility for addressing harms related to research.

Fortunately, the UK CHI models during the COVID pandemic also provide a potential solution to this challenge. The fact that this CHI research was done in a country with universal healthcare ensured that participants would have access to healthcare if they needed it years later. While universal healthcare is a key component of what participants might need in the future if they suffer long-term harm from research participation, a person who lost their job due to long COVID might also need a social safety net that can ensure they are able to support themselves even while unemployed. Thus, while many have considered the idea of setting up a fund to compensate injured research participants (Pike, 2012), it may also make sense to think about the government's role in determining access to healthcare and other forms of societal safety nets as a way to support the conduct of risky research. For harms that are realized years after a study has been conducted, social supports that are available to research participants might be the best way to ensure that they receive adequate compensation and do not bear the costs of their research-related injuries all on their own.

This analysis underscores the idea that site selection may be an important component of research ethics for studies beyond CHI research. While providing universal healthcare and social supports is an elegant potential solution to the problem of compensation for research-related injury, particularly if one thinks about the many countries that have already made investments in this regard, it becomes more challenging to address in others. For instance, countries like the United Kingdom and Norway would not have to invest much, if anything, more to support the ethical conduct of research that carries risks of long-term harms. On the other hand, countries like the United States and China would likely struggle to invest enough to build such an expensive solution to address the problem of long-term research-related injury, and they may face many structural and political hurdles to making such a change. Researchers who are agnostic about where to conduct studies with risks of long-term harms could select sites in countries that already have a strong social support network in place. Yet diverting risky research away from countries that do not have a strong social support network could also have many unintended consequences, including inefficiencies in terms of the failure to use existing research infrastructure as effectively as possible. While it would be hasty to conclude that risky research should only be done in countries with social supports in place, a surprising implication of this analysis of CHI research is that the need for compensation for longer-term harms from research provides yet another argument in support of universal healthcare and a social safety net. Furthermore, researchers should take into account the resources at a given site that would be available to help ensure the ethical conduct of research, including the ability to provide compensation for longer-term harms from research, when deciding where research should take place.

Self-Experimentation

Although self-experimentation has occurred in CHI research for centuries (Shah & Jamrozik E., 2020), the COVID-19 pandemic led to the rise of the advocacy group 1Day Sooner and, with it, a new way to think about self-experimentation. As noted in Chapter 1, in the early days of research ethics, self-experimentation was seen as a way to protect research participants. The Nuremberg Code included a provision that said that research in which high risks were likely to occur, specifically related to "death and disabling injury" should not be conducted, "except, perhaps, in those experiments where the experimental physicians also serve as subjects" (Nuremberg Military Tribunals, 1949). This provision was likely inserted as a way to rationalize that Walter Reed's yellow fever challenge trials were ethically appropriate despite the high risks involved (Miller & Joffe, 2009). During the COVID pandemic, 1Day Sooner had great success at building media interest and public support for the conduct of CHI research and has now moved on to funding the development of a Hepatitis C CHI model that can ultimately aid in the development of a Hepatitis C vaccine (Rid et al., 2023). 1Day Sooner's support of research raises questions about whether there should be some degree of increased legitimacy for, or decreased ethical scrutiny on, the prospect of exposing participants to high and uncertain risk. If patient or other advocacy groups are driving the research or even experimenting on themselves, this could change the ethical evaluation of research and permit more risky research to be conducted—but it may also raise different ethical concerns.

Alan Wertheimer and Frank Miller have argued that research regulation involves some degree of paternalism, which they conclude is primarily *soft paternalism* (Miller & Wertheimer, 2007). In other words, it is not that research oversight is necessarily designed to prevent people from participating in research for their own good—rather, the goal of regulation is to prevent people from enrolling in research they would not choose to engage in if they were fully informed. Miller and Wertheimer argue that research is difficult for laypeople to understand, and concerns about informed consent are typically rooted in the idea that people may not know what they are getting themselves into. Just as John Stuart Mill argued, it is acceptable to stop people from crossing over a bridge if they do not know that the bridge lacks structural integrity and poses great danger to them, so, too, can regulators build in informed consent requirements to ensure people understand the potential harms associated with research prior to enrolling in it. It is almost universally agreed that this form of justifiable soft paternalism should arguably have some place in all research, regardless of who funds or plans it.

On the other hand, *hard paternalism,* or preventing people from engaging in activities because of the idea that it is better for them not to engage, may have a very limited place in the regulation of research with adults who can consent when that research is conceived of, funded by, and participated in by the same people. This suggests that, if people engaging in self-experimentation are fully informed, there may be less justification for an upper limit of risk. Other ethical requirements might also need to be adjusted for research involving self-experimentation. For example, justifications for a social value requirement in research in part rely on the need for preserving public trust in research, maintaining researcher integrity, and spending research dollars responsibly (Wendler & Rid, 2017). These justifications may be less important when the same people are the ones making sure the research happens, are directly involved in planning the research, and when they put their own funds and/or bodies on the line. Thus, the surprising conclusion suggested from a closer examination of self-experimentation is that setting an upper limit of risk and enforcing a social value requirement might be less important for citizen science than for other types of research.

On the other hand, there might be other reasons that even self-experimentation should have social value. For example, some argue that research with limited social value (or value that only accrues to some groups rather than others) can exacerbate injustice (Wenner, 2017), which may be a relevant ethical consideration even for groups sponsoring research with their own funds. Additionally, self-experimentation may lead to situations where research has questionable social value if the assessment of social value is subject to conflicts of interest. The oversight and regulation of research is important in part because it is difficult to maintain objectivity about one's own projects (Emanuel et al., 2000). Overconfidence could lead projects to be conducted that have limited value, and the desire for one's projects to be successful could prevent participants in self-experimentation from reporting negative information about the symptoms they are experiencing (Shah & Jamrozik E., 2020). While these types of concerns might not rise to the level to make such research impermissible, they clearly suggest that self-experimentation should not be described as an ethical safeguard. Ultimately, self-experimentation may be more deserving of skepticism than celebration.

Elevating Research Participants

Research participants typically receive public attention when they have been harmed or exploited in research. Consider, for example, James Phipps, the 8-year-old famous for having been exposed to smallpox by Edward Jenner, or Jesse Gelsinger, who died in a gene therapy trial that was subject to substantial ethical criticism. The discussion of CHI research and the prominence of the advocacy organization 1DaySooner during the COVID-19 pandemic present an opportunity to rethink how research participants are conceived of by the general public. It could be incredibly valuable to decrease the stigma associated with research participation and promote greater societal respect for research participants and their contributions to science (Kraft et al., 2023).

Data suggest that participation in CHI research can be something that participants hide from others due to a fear of being teased or pressured not to participate (Kraft et al., 2019). Because the important contributions of research participants are typically not recognized by the general public and risks are often more salient, the fear of how others would react may dissuade some people from participating in research.

The generally unfavorable public impression of research participants is also a problem for people who argue that one way to tell if research risks are permissible is to compare them to other socially acceptable activities, or the so-called comparator method. This method has been used to argue that high-risk, high-value research should be permissible because it is similar to other activities that have social approval, such as humanitarian aid work or firefighting (Paquette & Shah, 2020). However, unlike the other examples where high risks are considered acceptable, research participants are not generally seen as heroic or worthy of respect from society. With only a few exceptions that prove the rule, most research participants who are widely known are those thought to have been exploited by researchers, such as Henrietta Lacks and Jesse Gelsinger. Research participants are often referred to as "guinea pigs" or "test bunnies"—terms that suggest a lack of agency and control. This suggests that, if high-risk research is to be ethically justifiable, more work is needed to change the public perception of research participants to more fully recognize their contributions to society and decrease the stigma associated with research participation (Kraft et al., 2023).

Conclusion

This chapter reveals that an in-depth analysis of CHI research can yield surprising insights for research ethics more generally. At the meta level, it is important to recognize that ethical issues should not be dismissed if they are not entirely unique. When new developments arise, more careful, all-things-considered judgments are needed that can address the combination of issues raised and the amount of existing guidance and resolution on them. This analysis of CHI research also has six other insights for research ethics more generally.

First, the "yuck" reaction, or intuitive sense that there is something wrong with a research study, is worth taking seriously for ethical and pragmatic reasons, particularly if members of the research team are experiencing it. Second, the fact that evaluating social value rigorously requires understanding the place of a particular study in a larger portfolio has two implications: (1) some studies may need more rigorous review of social value from expert actors by considering them in the context of larger research programs to which they belong, including sponsors and DMCs; and (2) it might be more fruitful for standard review, particularly of studies that pose low risks, to involve a limited check to determine whether the methods are likely to achieve a scientific aim that has promise. Third, the idea that it might be ethically acceptable to raise the upper limit of risk in an emergency fails to consider the deficiencies in decision-making that often arise in emergencies and the need for public trust. The COVID-19 pandemic revealed that speed can come at financial risk rather than risk to participants or public trust, and that even the perception of shortcuts can have long-term consequences for public trust. Fourth, site selection is more important ethically than has been realized, including when considering whether there is a social safety net in place that can provide participants with care if they experience longer-term harm from research. Fifth, self-experimentation is not a good way to justify risky research and raises clear concerns about objectivity and risk to those involved. However, it is not clear whether external actors can easily stand in judgment of research that is funded by and conducted with people who are so invested in the research without engaging in unjustified hard paternalism. Finally, CHI research illuminates the importance of elevating research participants' status in society. If research participants were given their due respect, rather than being recognized only when they are harmed or exploited, other questions in research ethics might be easier to answer, such as whether high-risk research should be permitted.

8

Lessons Learned About CHI
Research Ethics

*Q: What was your first reaction to the idea of a COVID-19
infection study?*
A: We are going in the direction of progress.
—Prospective volunteer for COVID-19 CHI research

In 2001, Frank Miller and Christine Grady launched a discussion among ethicists about controlled human infection (CHI) research. They acknowledged that their early assessment was a start of a conversation that would evolve over time, stating as follows: "In exploring the ethical justifiability of particular challenge experiments, it may be helpful to consider infection-inducing challenge models as falling along a continuum from those that are legitimate to those that are clearly unacceptable. . . . As the state of biomedical knowledge and treatment progresses, the location of possible challenge models along this spectrum is likely to shift" (Miller & Grady, 2001).

One key contribution of this book is to recognize that, in addition to the progress in biomedical knowledge and treatment that Miller and Grady anticipated, advances in bioethics have helped to facilitate CHI research. As our examination of the ethics of CHI research draws to a close, this final chapter is an opportunity to take stock of the progress made on the ethics of CHI research and its implications for research ethics in general. In this chapter, I summarize the larger lessons from this book and consider their implications for CHI research moving forward, identifying themes that span across this book.

Intentionally Infecting Humans. Seema K. Shah, Oxford University Press. © Seema K. Shah 2026.
DOI: 10.1093/9780197667927.003.0008

Summary of Ethics of CHI Research

There are several takeaways from this book for CHI research going forward. Perhaps most important is the recognition that CHI research is not wholly ethically distinct from other types of research although it can require extra ethical scrutiny. CHI research is unusual in that it raises a set of five complex and/or unresolved ethical issues all at once: (1) social value can be highly uncertain, (2) researchers intend to expose participants to illness, (3) participants can face high and uncertain risk of harm, (4) third parties may be exposed to risk, and 5), in some cases, early withdrawal from CHI research may be very risky for participants or third parties. Furthermore, when a new CHI model is being created, it has particularly high uncertainty in terms of its social value and risk. The process of developing a novel CHI model also sets the parameters for how key ethical issues will be addressed in future CHI studies. However, the common assumption that CHI research is distinct because it offers higher risks and financial rewards for research participants than other types of research is untrue.

Understanding the unusual aspects of CHI research, along with the difference between CHI models and CHI studies, reveals how ethical frameworks and oversight can be most effectively utilized. Existing ethical frameworks and guidelines for CHI research are valuable but need to be revised to clearly distinguish between the development of a CHI model from the use of an established model in CHI studies. The framework provided herein lays out eight criteria that have a higher burden of proof when applied to a new CHI model. Moreover, as a general rule, creating a new CHI model should include more procedural protections like specialized ethics review and engagement of interested parties. By contrast, when CHI studies are done with models that already have a track record of safety, they can typically use standard review processes, like Institutional Review Boards (IRBs). IRBs and their international equivalents can rely on the components of the framework and other guidance (World Health Organization, 2022).

The second major lesson is that the history of CHI research demonstrates its great potential for scientific progress along with its ethical challenges. While CHI research has been helpful to advance science, it has primarily been useful as a longer-term investment. It is also critically important to ensure that CHI research is conducted in a scientifically rigorous manner and under carefully controlled conditions designed to minimize risk. As we saw in Chapter 1, researchers who conducted challenge trials during the 1918 influenza pandemic injected patients with fluids from other patients who were thought to have influenza, making it unclear what participants were being given and what diseases they might contract (Jamrozik & Selgelid, 2020). This example and others like it led to ethical reform of CHI research, including a commitment to maintaining scientific integrity and conducting research in a controlled setting. Permitting CHI research that lacks rigor, caution in exposing participants to risk, or attention to the ethics would be a step backward, echoing the unethical research that was permitted in the past and failing to discharge the duties of researchers who are intentionally and directly exposing participants to pathogens.

Third, the ethically problematic behavior of challenge study researchers in the past still colors beliefs about research today and may also contribute to a "yuck" reaction to this research—an intuitive reaction that there must be something unethical about it (Kelly, 2011). Historical unethical research—both that which involved intentional infection and that which did not—continues to reverberate today and affects trust in research going forward. For example, it is not difficult to draw a line from the "ethically impossible" experiments conducted by the US government in Guatemala to modern-day concerns about decolonizing research in low- and middle-income countries (LMICs) (Abimbola & Pai, 2020). The egregious nature of the Tuskegee syphilis study is widely recognized but sometimes misunderstood. Many believe that the study involved deliberate infection, without realizing the unethical behavior of the researchers was to lie by omission and withhold a cure for syphilis from participants over decades, exposing not only the participants but also their families to substantial risk in the process (Scharff et al., 2010). Nazi experiments infecting people who were incarcerated in concentration camps are an especially important example of how the "yuck" reaction may be activated by historical examples of unethical challenge studies, particularly in light of the evidence suggesting that a sweater worn by Adolf Hitler provoked the strongest "yuck" reaction out of all of the potentially disgusting stimuli used by a group of experimental psychologists (Kelly, 2011).

While the "yuck" reaction may serve as a valuable signal for ethical concern in CHI research, it is hardly sufficient to identify whether there is real cause for concern, and it sometimes misfires badly. The fact that the "yuck" reaction is likely based in an evolutionary response to disgust is borne out by the recognition that different types of CHI research can provoke different levels of reactions (Kelly, 2011). For example, the "yuck" reaction seems to be intuitively triggered more by CHI research that infects people by having them drink a solution filled with parasitic worms than by exposing them to influenza, even though influenza CHI research is higher risk. However, the fact that some CHI research raises a greater "yuck" reaction than other types is worth paying attention to when considering potential public reactions to such research and the need for community engagement in advance. Approaches to community engagement in CHI research should be informed by the likely responses of members of the public. If CHI research is likely to include a "yuck reaction" for some reason, researchers could plan more intensive educational interventions for potential participants and better engagement with members of the public and also make space to address ethical concerns harbored by people serving on study teams who might be reluctant to raise their concerns but face challenges in carrying out the research if these concerns remain unaddressed.

Fourth, CHI research was overhyped in the COVID-19 pandemic but could be of value in future pandemic preparedness as a longer-term proposition. Taking a closer look at whether CHI research was useful in the Zika and COVID-19 pandemics revealed great promise along with possibilities that were always unlikely to be realized. While some have argued that CHI research was delayed by unnecessary ethical caution, it took just as long to develop the first CHI model, even under highly favorable circumstances, as it did to run three phases of trials to test vaccines that were accelerated by taking financial risks. The COVID-19 pandemic revealed that when field trials can be done rapidly, CHI research is not a great alternative for testing vaccines and treatments (Grady et al., 2020). More generally, CHI research should be thought of as a complement to other types of research, not a standalone method for testing vaccines. While speeding up some components of CHI research is clearly worth pursuing, including considering whether ensuring quality control of CHI research (e.g., through the use of adapted procedures to strain and purify infectious agents) can use specialized processes rather than borrowing them from other areas, there is a danger to some suggestions that focus on speed as the main consideration. For instance, calls to rely more heavily on "natural exposure" CHI models fail to acknowledge that these models may be well-suited to answering some questions and not others and also pay insufficient attention to the additional challenges involved, including the fact that the variability in how likely different people are to infect others may make it very difficult to develop a model for some diseases in this way (Eyal & Lipsitch, 2021).

Furthermore, it seems clear that CHI research may not be the most useful in the early stages of a public health emergency, when very little is known about the spreading pathogen. Indeed, the meteoric rise in ethical attention to CHI research during the COVID-19 pandemic may have done a disservice to this research method. The hype surrounding CHI research overshadowed its many potential contributions and made it less clear how to use it effectively. The Zika epidemic demonstrated that CHI research can be a useful back-up to field trials if transmission of a pathogen becomes unpredictable but the pathogen remains a threat (Vannice et al., 2019). Another promising potential use of CHI research during pandemics is to develop or deploy models of viruses that are related to pathogens that have pandemic potential but pose much lower risk (Halstead, 2020). During the COVID-19 pandemic, information from CHI models of cold-inducing coronaviruses that were much milder than SARS-CoV-2 was useful for understanding transmission and the likely course of infection. CHI research can be a valuable way to build knowledge about a diverse family of pathogens, some of which generally cause mild symptoms and others of which can bring the world to a halt. Instead of thinking of CHI research as a silver bullet to use in case of an emergency, it may be more helpful to conceive of CHI research as a longer-term investment in understanding infectious diseases with pandemic potential.

Perhaps more fundamentally, it may be helpful to rethink the amount of energy that was spent on CHI research during the COVID-19 pandemic. Consider that more than 38,000 people volunteered to be deliberately infected with a virus about which little was known and that several academics, myself included, contributed their time and energy to the US government and the World Health Organization to rapidly produce the guidance documents and infrastructure support. The quick mobilization of so many groups of people around CHI research is laudable, but it might have been better if that energy had been devoted to other types of research, such as vaccine studies or treatment trials. The COVID-19 pandemic also revealed important and understudied challenges, such as the need to bolster public trust, decrease vaccine hesitancy, and attend to the off-target effects of public health interventions, such as the exacerbation of an ongoing pediatric mental health crisis by school closures.

A fifth takeaway from this book is that, as CHI research expands into new populations, a cautious approach is advisable—but blanket exclusion is not. As illustrated by recent guidance for CHI research developed in Kenya and India, the expansion of CHI research requires strong justification, broad consultation, and the application of rigorous ethical conditions. Furthermore, the distinction between CHI models and CHI studies makes clear that not all CHI research is created equal, and this guidance would do well to make the distinction sharper in terms of where they start and how their review systems are structured. Perhaps most importantly, countries beginning new programs of CHI research should take care to start with studies that use established models with a solid track record of safety.

There are several examples of low-risk or even beneficial CHI studies, including the use of CHI research with benign, beneficial bacteria that can prevent infection from disease-causing bacteria (akin to taking probiotics) (Theodosiou et al., 2022). This suggests that there is considerable room for expansion of lower-risk CHI research to build greater capacity around the world. While there may not be an ethical imperative to expand CHI research, it is important to recognize the potential added value of CHI research in addressing long-neglected diseases. The field of global health has long had a myopic approach to determining what counts as most important. Many pathogens have created conditions that could be thought of as emergencies, but because they have afflicted people in LMICs, they have received little attention elsewhere. CHI research may be an important way to make progress on diseases that have been neglected because they are experienced mostly by people in LMICs, provided this research is held to rigorous ethical standards and with attention to the importance of decolonizing global health. When the goal of CHI research on a neglected disease is to address prior injustices, leadership from LMIC researchers and engagement with communities are critical to ensure that the CHI research is actually a priority for those most affected by the disease. Furthermore, inclusion of participants from groups with a history of exclusion from research because of their perceived vulnerability can be important as a matter of justice. Inclusion of these groups can and should start with lower-risk CHI research and the development of tailored protections to address the specific ways in which participants could be wronged or harmed.

Finally, by subjecting CHI research to a sustained ethical analysis, this book has revealed several implications for research ethics more generally. First, the intuitive ethical concern that members of the public or members of research teams might feel is important to address because it may reveal ethical issues that went unnoticed or qualms that are not based on real moral concern but could hamper the research if left unchecked. Second, understanding the social value of research often requires appreciating a trial as one part of a research portfolio, contrary to how our research ethics system conducts oversight. This can be addressed through more careful review of social value outside of the IRB system, such as by research sponsors or Data Monitoring Committees. Yet this also could free up IRBs to focus less on social value in some cases. Because it is difficult to accurately evaluate social value and unnecessary to have precision in measuring social value for low-risk research that does not need compelling value to justify it, IRBs and their international equivalents may be able to judge simply whether the social value of a given study crosses the threshold of acceptability. For example, IRBs could engage in a quick calculation of whether the methods are likely to answer an important question that has not already been asked and answered many times over.

A third implication of this analysis relates to debates about the upper limit of risk of research that have suggested that it might be ethically acceptable to exceed standard risk limits in an emergency. As the COVID-19 pandemic revealed, even the perception of shortcuts can have long-term consequences for public trust. Moreover, decision-making in the heat of a pandemic was not always sound, casting doubt on whether it would be wise to abandon ethical limits for research in emergencies. A fourth implication is that *where* research is conducted matters morally, especially if certain sites offer national health insurance and social safety nets that can protect participants from longer-term harms that materialize long after the research is over. This analysis of CHI research has also revealed that self-experimentation (i.e., having researchers and sponsors participate as subjects in their own research) can raise concerns about objectivity, value, and risk—but also that research that is funded by and conducted with the same people is difficult to criticize without lapsing into unjustified paternalism. Finally, one of the enduring lessons of this book is how much of scientific progress depends on people who are willing to take on risk for the benefit of others. It is critically important to make progress on developing ways to demonstrate respect to research participants from others in society, rather than accepting the benefits that come from research and paying attention to those who take on the burdens only when they are harmed or exploited.

Future Horizons for CHI Research and Research Ethics

This analysis of the ethics of CHI research has also revealed several issues that would benefit from more research. First, the risks associated with research are not reported in the literature as well as is necessary to thoroughly evaluate different types of research. This failure to fully report safety of CHI research poses challenges for determining whether this research is ethically acceptable and how best to regulate it, and it should be addressed. While existing data suggest that CHI research can be conducted safely and poses a wide range of risk and uncertainty depending on the pathogen and model being used, there is an urgent need for more rigorous data collection about the risks of these studies, particularly regarding third parties. For example, in Chapter 3, we saw that one-third of all CHI research reported in the literature did not report any adverse events that participants experienced (Adams-Phipps et al., 2022). Additionally, one experience commonly discussed at scientific meetings involves a participant in a CHI study who left the country after having been infected with malaria; this person had to be tracked down by international legal authorities to ensure they received treatment and did not infect others, and this incident has never been reported in the literature to my knowledge (Richie, 2019). There is also an ongoing debate about whether a challenge study conducted in the 1970s led to a global influenza epidemic, and this possible harm is not typically cited in literature reviewing the safety of CHI research (Rozo & Gronvall, 2015). There is similar underreporting for Phase I trials with healthy volunteers (Johnson et al., 2016). These gaps in knowledge make it difficult to know how risky CHI research is and how to compare it to other types of research.

A second issue related to CHI research is how to measure and consider public trust. Attempts to measure public trust in CHI research may be subject to serious limitations. One study of international support for CHI research described such research as likely to make vaccines for COVID-19 available sooner than standard methods, which was not the case (Broockman et al., 2021). This flawed premise makes it difficult to interpret the findings. A different study of stakeholders in India found a great deal of skepticism about CHI research and concerns about whether it could ever be ethical to do such work based on a perception of a long history of unethical research in India (Vaz et al., 2021). Yet measuring public attitudes in a country with so much diversity requires drilling down into the views of different groups of people, including those likely to be approached for enrollment into CHI research. Additionally, the "yuck" factor, common misconceptions about CHI research, and challenges in explaining key distinctions such as the difference between models and studies all may need to be a part of educational efforts about this type of research before soliciting opinions on whether it should be conducted. This suggests that more research is needed on public perceptions of CHI research, but that it may be important to measure baseline perceptions of

CHI research along with what members of the public think about this type of research after receiving education about the research method.

Finally, how to communicate about and encourage longer-term investments in scientific advancement and pandemic preparedness is an important challenge. If the insight that CHI research should generally be a longer-term investment dampens enthusiasm for this research, that may be short-sighted. Members of the public, including the media, may need help connecting the dots between different types of research that, over time, build into a deep understanding of science that can lead to new insights and interventions that can suddenly become essential when disaster strikes.

Conclusion

When the next pandemic strikes, it would be ideal to have a foundation to build on to avoid the deficiencies of the past. Furthermore, many threats to well-being may move more slowly or insidiously than pandemics but still deserve our attention. Ultimately, my hope is that this book makes sufficient progress on the ethics of CHI research to facilitate better decision-making about when to turn to this research method—and when not to—to help solve the many public health problems likely to arise in the future.

References

1Day Sooner. (2020). Volunteer for high-impact challenge trials. Retrieved from https://1daysooner.org/

1Day Sooner. (2024). Using challenge trials in public health emergencies: A roundtable discussion. https://www.1daysooner.org/1day-sooner-hosts-rou ndtable-on-human-challenge-studies-during-emerging-health-emergencies/

Aaronson, S., Ahuja, A., Anderson, C., Berger, A., Caplan, A., Eyal, N., Glassman, J., Krawiec, K., Lipsitch, M., Marsh, A., Morrison, J., Plotkin, S., Rose, S., Rouphael, N., Satel, S., Singer, P., Wharton, K., Wikler, D., Capecchi, M., . . . Zuckerman D. (2020, July 15). US: Challenge trials for COVID-19 [Open Letter]. Retrieved from https://www.1daysooner.org/us-open-letter/

Abimbola, S., & Pai, M. (2020). Will global health survive its decolonisation? The Lancet (British edition), 396(10263), 1627–1628. https://doi.org/10.1016/S0140-6736(20)32417-X

Abo, Y.-N., Jamrozik, E., McCarthy, J. S., Roestenberg, M., Steer, A. C., & Osowicki, J. (2023). Strategic and scientific contributions of human challenge trials for vaccine development: Facts versus fantasy. The Lancet Infectious Diseases, 23(12), e533–e546. https://doi.org/10.1016/S1473-3099(23)00294-3

Academy of Medical Sciences. (2005). Microbial challenge studies of human volunteers. Retrieved from https://acmedsci.ac.uk/file-download/34726-112 7728424.pdf

Academy of Medical Sciences. (2018). Controlled human infection model studies: Summary of a workshop held on 6 February 2018. Retrieved from https://acmedsci.ac.uk/policy/policy-projects/controlled-human-infection-models

Adams-Phipps, J., Toomey, D., Wiecek, W., Schmit, V., Wilkinson, J., Scholl, K., Jamrozik, E., Osowicki, J., Roestenberg, M., & Manheim, D. (2023). A systematic review of human challenge trials, designs, and safety. Clinical Infectious Disease, 76(4), 609–619. https://doi.org/10.1093/cid/ciac820

American Academy of Pediatrics Committee on Nutrition. (2000). Hypoallergenic infant formulas. Pediatrics (Evanston), 106(2 Pt 1), 346–349.

Anomaly, J., & Savulescu, J. (2019). Compensation for cures: Why we should pay a premium for participation in 'challenge studies'. Bioethics, 33(7), 792–797. https://onlinelibrary.wiley.com/doi/full/10.1111/bioe.12596

Anywaine, Z., Lule, S. A., Hansen, C., Warimwe, G., & Elliott, A. (2022). Clinical manifestations of Rift Valley fever in humans: Systematic review and meta-analysis. PLoS Neglected Tropical Disease, 16(3), e0010233. https://doi.org/10.1371/journal.pntd.0010233

Association of American Physicians. (1898). Transactions of the Association of American Physicians. W. J. Dornan. Retrieved from https://books.google.com/books?id=qZVIAAAAYAAJ

Austin, S. C., Stolley, P. D., & Lasky, T. (1992). The history of malariotherapy for neurosyphilis: Modern parallels. *Journal of the American Medical Association*, *268*(4), 516–519. https://do:.org/10.1001/jama.1992.03490040092031

Baay, M., & Neels, P. (2020). SARS-CoV-2 controlled human infection models: Ethics, challenge agent production and regulatory issues. *Biologicals*, *67*, 69–74. https://doi.org/10.1016/j.biologicals.2020.08.006

Baay, M. F. D., Richie, T. L., Neels, P., & Session chairs at the second Human Challenge Trials, m. (2019). Human challenge trials in vaccine development, Rockville, MD, USA, September 28–30, 2017. *Biologicals*, *61*, 85–94. https://doi. org/10.1016/j.biologicals.2018.02.002

Bambery, B., Selgelid, M., Weijer, C., Savulescu, J., & Pollard, A. J. (2016). Ethical criteria for human challenge studies in infectious diseases. *Public Health Ethics*, *9*(1), 92–103. https://doi.org/10.1093/phe/phv026

Barker, C., Collet, K., Gbesemete, D., Piggin, M., Watson, D., Pristera, P., Lawerence, W., Smith, C., Bahrami-Hessari, M., Johnson, H., Baker, K., Qavi, A., McGrath, C., Chiu, C., Read, R. C., & Ward, H. (2022). Public attitudes to a human challenge study with SARS-CoV-2: A mixed-methods study. *Wellcome Open Research*, *7*, 49. https://doi.org/10.12688/wellcomeopenres.17516.1

Barnes, M. V. C., Mandla, A., Smith, E., Maskuniitty, M., & Openshaw, P. J. M. (2023). Human infection challenge in the pandemic era and beyond, HIC-Vac annual meeting report, 2022. *Immunotherapy Advances*, *3*(1), ltad024–ltad024. https://doi.org/10.1093/immadv/ltad024

Barnhill, A., Joffe, S., & Miller, F. G. (2016). The ethics of infection challenges in primates. *Hastings Center Report*, *46*(4), 20–26. https://doi.org/10.1002/hast.580

Bastiaens, G. J. H., van Meer, M. P. A., Scholzen, A., Obiero, J. M., Vatanshenassan, M., van Grinsven, T., Sim, B. K. L., Billingsley, P. F., James, E. R., Gunasekera, A., Bijker, E. M., van Gemert, G. J., van de Vegte-Bolmer, M., Graumans, W., Hermsen, C. C., de Mast, Q., van der Ven, A., Hoffman, S. L., & Sauerwein, R. W. (2016). Safety, immunogenicity, and protective efficacy of intradermal immunization with aseptic, purified, cryopreserved Plasmodium falciparum sporozoites in volunteers under chloroquine prophylaxis: A randomized controlled trial. *American Journal of Tropical Medicine and Hygiene*, *4*(3), 663–673. https://doi.org/10.4269/ajtmh.15-0621

Baumgaertner, E. (April 24, 2018). Ethicists call for more scrutiny of "human-challenge" trials. *New York Times*, Section D, 3. Retrieved from https://www.nytimes.com/2018/04/20/health/zika-study-ethics.html

Baxby, D. (1985). The genesis of Edward Jenner's Inquiry of 1798: A comparison of the two unpublished manuscripts and the published version. *Medical History*, *29*(2), 193–199. https://doi.org/10.1017/S0025727300044008

Bearcroft, W. (1956). Zika virus infection experimentally induced in a human volunteer. *Transactions of the Royal Society of Tropical Medicine and Hygiene*, *50*(5), 442–448. https://doi.org/10.1016/0035-9203(56)90091-8

Beecher, H. K. (1966). Ethics and clinical research. *New England Journal of Medicine*, *274*(24), 1354–1360. https://doi.org/10.1056/NEJM196606162742405

Belshe, R. B., & Van Voris, L. P. (1984). Cold-recombinant influenza A/California/10/78 (H1N1) virus vaccine (CR-37) in seronegative children: Infectivity and efficacy against investigational challenge. *Journal of Infectious Diseases, 149*(5), 735–740. https://doi.org/10.1093/infdis/149.5.735

Bennett, J. W., Pybus, B. S., Yadava, A., Tosh, D., Sousa, J. C., McCarthy, W. F., Deye, G., Melendez, V., & Ockenhouse, C. F. (2013). Primaquine failure and cytochrome p-450 2D6 in *Plasmodium vivax* malaria. *New England Journal of Medicine, 369*(14), 1381–1382. https://doi.org/doi:10.1056/NEJMc1301936

Bennett, J. W., Yadava, A., Tosh, D., Sattabongkot, J., Komisar, J., Ware, L. A., McCarthy, W. F., Cowden, J. J., Regules, J., Spring, M. D., Paolino, K., Hartzell, J. D., Cummings, J. F., Richie, T. L., Lumsden, J., Kamau, E., Murphy, J., Lee, C., Parekh, F., . . . Ockenhouse, C. F. (2016). Phase 1/2a trial of Plasmodium vivax malaria vaccine candidate VMP001/AS01 B in malaria-naive adults: Safety, immunogenicity, and efficacy: E0004423. *PLoS Neglected Tropical Diseases, 10*(2), e0004423. https://doi.org/https://doi.org/10.1371/journal.pntd.0004423

Bennett, S. (2020). Pfizer and Moderna Covid vaccines 95% effective in clinical trials. Retrieved from https://www.pbs.org/wgbh/nova/article/pfizer-mode rna-covid-vaccines-clinical-trials/

Benyajati, C. (1966). Experimental cholera in humans. *British Medical Journal, 1*(5480), 140–142. https://doi.org/10.1136/bmj.1.5480.140

Bernkopf, H., Treu, G., & Maythar, B. (1964). Human infection experiments with three cell-cultured trachoma agents. *Archives of Ophthalmology (1960), 71*(5), 693–700. https://doi.org/10.1001/archopht.1964.00970010709018

Bernstein, D. I., Atmar, R. L., Lyon, G. M., Treanor, J. J., Chen, W. H., Jiang, X., Vinje, J., Gregoricus, N., Frenck, R. W., Jr., Moe, C. L., Al-Ibrahim, M. S., Barrett, J., Ferreira, J., Estes, M. K., Graham, D. Y., Goodwin, R., Borkowski, A., Clemens, R., & Mendelman, P. M. (2015). Norovirus vaccine against experimental human GII.4 virus illness: A challenge study in healthy adults. *Journal of Infectious Disease, 211*(6), 870–878. https://doi.org/10.1093/infdis/jiu497

Binik, A. (2024). Should children be included in human challenge studies? *Ethics & Human Research, 46*(3), 2–15. https://doi.org/10.1002/eahr.500208

Bos, W., Westra, A., de Beaufort, I., & van de Vathorst, S. (2017). To stop or not to stop: Dissent and undue burden as reasons to stop participation in paediatric research. *Journal of Medical Ethics, 43*(8), 519–523. https://doi.org/10.1136/medethics-2016-103788

Branswell, H. (2017). Ethics panel blocks proposed Zika vaccine research. *STAT News*. Retrieved from https://www.statnews.com/2017/02/28/zika-vaccine-eth ics-panel/

Brazil National Council of Health. (2012). Guidelines and rules for research involving human subjects. Resolution n° 466, December 12, 2012, Brasília. Retrieved from https://clinregs.niaid.nih.gov/sites/default/files/documents/brazil/ResNo466_GoogleTranslate.pdf

Brickley, E. B., Strauch, C. B., Wieland-Alter, W. F., Connor, R. I., Lin, S., Weiner, J. A., Ackerman, M. E., Arita, M., Oberste, M. S., Weldon, W. C., Sáez-Llorens, X., Bandyopadhyay, A. S., & Wright, P. F. (2018). Intestinal immune responses to type 2 oral polio vaccine (OPV) challenge in infants previously immunized with bivalent OPV and either high-dose or standard inactivated polio vaccine. *Journal of Infectious Diseases, 217*(3), 371–380. https://doi.org/10.1093/infdis/jix556

Broockman, D., Kalla, J., Guerrero, A., Budolfson, M., Eyal, N., Jewell, N. P., Magalhaes, M., & Sekhon, J. S. (2021). Broad cross-national public support for accelerated COVID-19 vaccine trial designs. *Vaccine, 39*(2), 309–316. https://doi.org/10.1016/j.vaccine.2020.11.072

Calina, D., Hartung, T., Docea, A. O., Spandidos, D. A., Egorov, A. M., Shtilman, M. I., Carvalho, F., & Tsatsakis, A. (2020). COVID-19 vaccines: Ethical framework concerning human challenge studies. *DARU Journal of Pharmaceutical Sciences, 28*(2), 807–812. https://doi.org/10.1007/s40 199-020-00371-8

Callaway, E. (2024). Scientists tried to give people COVID – and failed. *Nature (London),629*(8011),269–270. https://doi.org/10.1038/d41586-024-01284-1

Callow, K. A., Parry, H. F., Sergeant, M., & Tyrrell, D. A. (1990). The time course of the immune response to experimental coronavirus infection of man. *Epidemiology & Infection, 105*(2), 435–446. https://doi.org/10.1017/s09502 68800048019

Carabelli, A. M., Peacock, T. P., Thorne, L. G., Harvey, W. T., Hughes, J., de Silva, T. I., Peacock, S. J., Barclay, W. S., de Silva, T. I., Towers, G. J., Robertson, D. L., & Consortium, C.-G. U. (2023). SARS-CoV-2 variant biology: Immune escape, transmission and fitness. *Nature Reviews Microbiology, 21*(3), 162–177. https://doi.org/10.1038/s41579-022-00841-7

Cauchemez, S. D., Besnard, M. M. D., Bompard, P. M. P. H., Dub, T. M. P. H., Guillemette-Artur, P. M. D., Eyrolle-Guignot, D. M. D., Salje, H. P., Van Kerkhove, M. D. P., Abadie, V. P., Garel, C. M. D., Fontanet, A. P., & Mallet, H.-P. M. D. (2016). Association between Zika virus and microcephaly in French Polynesia, 2013–15: A retrospective study. *Lancet, 387*(10033), 2125–2132. https://doi.org/10.1016/S0140-6736(16)00651-6

Centers for Disease Control. (2023). CDC museum COVID-19 timeline. Retrieved from https://www.cdc.gov/museum/timeline/covid19.html

Centers for Disease Control and Prevention. (2024). Chickenpox (Varicella). Retrieved from https://www.cdc.gov/chickenpox/about/index.html#:~:text= CDC%20strongly%20recommends%20against%20hosting,death%2C%20e ven%20in%20healthy%20children

Charash, M., & McKay, D. (2002). Attention bias for disgust. *Journal of Anxiety Disorders, 16*(5), 529–541. https://doi.org/https://doi.org/10.1016/ S0887-6185(02)00171-8

Chaves-Carballo, E. (2013). Clara Maass, yellow fever and human experimentation. *Military Medicine, 178*(5), 557–562. https://doi.org/10.7205/MIL MED-D-12-00430

Chi, P. C., Owino, E. A., Jao, I., Bejon, P., Kapulu, M., Marsh, V., & Kamuya, D. (2022). Ethical considerations around volunteer payments in a malaria human infection study in Kenya: An embedded empirical ethics study. *BMC Medical Ethics, 23*(46), 1–13. https://doi.org/10.1186/s12910-022-00783-y

Chwang, E. (2008). Against the inalienable right to withdraw from research. *Bioethics, 22*(7), 370–378. https://doi.org/10.1111/j.1467-8519.2008.00666.x

Cohen Jr., M. M. (2010). Overview of German, Nazi, and Holocaust medicine. *American Journal of Medical Genetics Part A, 152A*(3), 687–707. https://doi.org/ https://doi.org/10.1002/ajmg.a.32807

Cohen, S., Doyle, W. J., Alper, C. M., Janicki-Deverts, D., & Turner, R. B. (1960/2009). Sleep habits and susceptibility to the common cold. *Archives of Internal Medicine, 169*(1), 62–67. https://doi.org/10.1001/archinternmed.2008.505

Comber, L., O Murchu, E., Drummond, L., Carty, P. G., Walsh, K. A., De Gascun, C. F., Connolly, M. A., Smith, S. M., O'Neill, M., Ryan, M., & Harrington, P. (2021). Airborne transmission of SARS-CoV-2 via aerosols. *Reviews in Medical Virology, 31*(3), e2184–n/a. https://doi.org/10.1002/rmv.2184

Consumer News and Business Channel. (2020). Moderna CEO reportedly expects coronavirus vaccine interim results in November. Retrieved from https://www.cnbc.com/2020/10/20/moderna-ceo-reportedly-expects-coronavirus-vaccine-interim-results-in-november.html

Cornwall, W. (2020). New challenges emerge for planned human challenge trials. *Science, 370*(6521), 1150–1150. https://doi.org/doi:10.1126/science.370.6521.1150

Council for International Organizations of Medical Sciences. (2016). International ethical guidelines for health-related research involving humans. World Health Organization. Retrieved from https://cioms.ch/wp-content/uploads/2017/01/WEB-CIOMS-EthicalGuidelines.pdf

Council of Europe. (2005). Additional protocol to the Convention on Human Rights and Biomedicine, concerning biomedical research. Retrieved from https://rm.coe.int/168008371a

Creinin, M. D., Hou, M. Y., Dalton, L., Steward, R., & Chen, M. J. (2020). Mifepristone antagonization with progesterone to prevent medical abortion: A randomized controlled trial. *Obstetrics and Gynecology, 135*(1), 158–165. https://doi.org/10.1097/AOG.0000000000003620

Crook, H., Raza, S., Nowell, J., Young, M., & Edison, P. (2021). Long COVID: Mechanisms, risk factors, and management. *BMJ (Online), 374,* n1648–n1648. https://doi.org/10.1136/bmj.n1648

Cryder, C. E., John London, A., Volpp, K. G., & Loewenstein, G. (2010). Informative inducement: Study payment as a signal of risk. *Social Science & Medicine (1982), 70*(3), 455–464. https://doi.org/10.1016/j.socscimed.2009.10.047

Dabira, E. D., Fehr, A., Beloum, N., Van Geertruyden, J.-P., Achan, J., Erhart, A., Martinez-Alvarez, M., & D'Alessandro, U. (2023). Perceptions and acceptability of the controlled human malaria infection (CHMI) model in The Gambia: A qualitative study. *Scientific Reports, 13*(1), 8708–8708. https://doi.org/10.1038/s41598-023-35752-x

Dahlin, E., Nelson, G. M., Haynes, M., & Sargeant, F. (2016). Success rates for product development strategies in new drug development. *Journal of Clinical Pharmacy Therapy, 41*(2), 198–202. https://doi.org/10.1111/jcpt.12362

Dale, A. P., Gbesemete, D. F., Read, R. C., & Laver, J. R. (2022). Neisseria lactamica controlled human infection model. *Bacterial Vaccines, 2414,* 387–404. https://doi.org/10.1007/978-1-0716-1900-1_21

Darwin, C. (1872). Disdain, contempt, disgust, pride, etc., Helplessness, patience, affirmation and negation. In C. Darwin (Ed.), *The expression of the emotions in man and animals* (pp. 253–277). D. Appleton & Company.

Davies, H. (2007). Ethical reflections on Edward Jenner's experimental treatment. *Journal of Medical Ethics, 33*(3), 174–176. https://doi.org/10.1136/jme.2005.015339

Davies, H. (2023). UK Research Ethics Committee's review of the global first SARS-CoV-2 human infection challenge studies. *Journal of Medical Ethics, 49*(5), 322–324. https://doi.org/10.1136/medethics-2021-107709

Deasy, A. M., Guccione, E., Dale, A. P., Andrews, N., Evans, C. M., Bennett, J. S., Bratcher, H. B., Maiden, M. C., Gorringe, A. R., & Read, R. C. (2015). Nasal inoculation of the commensal Neisseria lactamica inhibits carriage of Neisseria meningitidis by young adults: A controlled human infection study. *Clinical Infectious Disease, 60*(10), 1512–1520. https://doi.org/10.1093/cid/civ098

DeGrazia, D., & Miller, F. G. (2021). Severe acute respiratory syndrome coronavirus 2 (SARS-CoV-2) infection challenge experiments in nonhuman primates: An ethical perspective. *Clinical Infectious Diseases, 73*(11), 2121–2125. https://doi.org/10.1093/cid/ciab278

de Jong, S. E., van Unen, V., Manurung, M. D., Stam, K. A., Goeman, J. J., Jochems, S. P., Höllt, T., Pezzotti, N., Mouwenda, Y. D., Betouke Ongwe, M. E., Lorenz, F.-R., Kruize, Y. C. M., Azimi, S., König, M. H., Vilanova, A., Eisemann, E., Lelieveldt, B. P. F., Roestenberg, M., Sim, B. K. L., ... Yazdanbakhsh, M. (2021). Systems analysis and controlled malaria infection in Europeans and Africans elucidate naturally acquired immunity. *Nature Immunology, 22*(5), 654–665. https://doi.org/10.1038/s41590-021-00911-7

Deming, M. E., Michael, N. L., Robb, M., Cohen, M. S., & Neuzil, K. M. (2020). Accelerating development of SARS-CoV-2 vaccines: The role for controlled human infection models. *New England Journal of Medicine, 383*(10), e63. https://doi.org/10.1056/NEJMp2020076

Deng, W., Bao, L., Gao, H., Xiang, Z., Qu, Y., Song, Z., Gong, S., Liu, J., Liu, J., Yu, P., Qi, F., Xu, Y., Li, F., Xiao, C., Lv, Q., Xue, J., Wei, Q., Liu, M., Wang, G., ... Qin, C. (2020). Ocular conjunctival inoculation of SARS-CoV-2 can cause mild COVID-19 in rhesus macaques. *Nature Communications, 11*(1), 4400–4400. https://doi.org/10.1038/s41467–020-18149–6

Denny, C. C., & Grady, C. (2007). Clinical research with economically disadvantaged populations. *Journal of Medical Ethics, 33*(7), 382–385. https://doi.org/10.1136/jme.2006.017681

Desilver, D. (2021). The U.S. differs from most other countries in how it sets its minimum wage. Pew Research Center. Retrieved from https://www.pewresearch.org/short-reads/2021/05/20/the-u-s-differs-from-most-other-countries-in-how-it-sets-its-minimum-wage/

DeVita, M. A., Wicclair, M., Swanson, D., Valenta, C., Schold, C., Ethics Committee, U. P. H., & Committee for the Oversight of Research Involving the Dead, U. o. P. (2003). Research involving the newly dead: An institutional response. *Critical Care Medicine, 31*(5 Suppl), S385–390. https://doi.org/10.1097/01.CCM.0000065142.41379.5C

Dhanani, L. Y., & Franz, B. (2022). A meta-analysis of COVID-19 vaccine attitudes and demographic characteristics in the United States. *Public Health (London), 207*, 31–38. https://doi.org/10.1016/j.puhe.2022.03.012

Dick, G. W. A., Kitchen, S. F., & Haddow, A. J. (1952). Zika Virus (I). Isolations and serological specificity. *Transactions of the Royal Society of Tropical Medicine and Hygiene, 46*(5), 509–520. https://doi.org/10.1016/0035–9203(52)90042–4

Dickert, N., & Grady, C. (1999). What's the price of a research subject? Approaches to payment for research participation. *New England Journal of Medicine, 341*(3), 198–203. https://doi.org/10.1056/NEJM199907153410312

Dorey, R. B., Theodosiou, A. A., Read, R. C., Vandrevala, T., & Jones, C. E. (2023). Qualitative interview study exploring the perspectives of pregnant women on participating in controlled human infection research in the UK. *BMJ Open*, *13*(12), e073992–e073992. https://doi.org/10.1136/bmjopen-2023-073992

Dube, K., Kanazawa, J., Taylor, J., Dee, L., Jones, N., Roebuck, C., Sylla, L., Louella, M., Kosmyna, J., Kelly, D., Clanton, O., Palm, D., Campbell, D. M., Onaiwu, M. G., Patel, H., Ndukwe, S., Henley, L., Johnson, M. O., Saberi, P., . . . Sugarman, J. (2021). Ethics of HIV cure research: An unfinished agenda. *BMC Medical Ethics*, *22*(1), 83. https://doi.org/10.1186/s12910-021-00651-1

Duffy, M. R., Chen, T.-H., Hancock, W. T., Powers, A. M., Kool, J. L., Lanciotti, R. S., Pretrick, M., Marfel, M., Holzbauer, S., Dubray, C., Guillaumot, L., Griggs, A., Bel, M., Lambert, A. J., Laven, J., Kosoy, O., Panella, A., Biggerstaff, B. J., Fischer, M., & Hayes, E. B. (2009). Zika virus outbreak on Yap Island, Federated States of Micronesia. *New England Journal of Medicine*, *360*(24), 2536–2543. https://doi.org/10.1056/NEJMoa0805715

Durbin, A. P., & Whitehead, S. S. (2017). Zika vaccines: Role for controlled human infection. *Journal of Infectious Diseases*, *216*(Suppl 10), S971–S975. https://doi.org/10.1093/infdis/jix491

Du Toit, G., Roberts, G., Sayre, P. H., Bahnson, H. T., Radulovic, S., Santos, A. F., Brough, H. A., Phippard, D., Basting, M., Feeney, M., Turcanu, V., Sever, M. L., Gomez Lorenzo, M., Plaut, M., & Lack, G. (2015). Randomized trial of peanut consumption in infants at risk for peanut allergy. *New England Journal of Medicine*, *372*(9), 803–813.

Dwyer C. (2020). Moderna's COVID-19 vaccine becomes 2nd to earn FDA authorization. *NPR*. Retrieved from https://www.npr.org/sections/coronavirus-live-updates/2020/12/18/947948227/modernas-covid-19-vaccine-becomes-2nd-to-earn-fda-authorization

Edwards, D. A., Ausiello, D., Salzman, J., Devlin, T., Langer, R., Beddingfield, B. J., Fears, A. C., Doyle-Meyers, L. A., Redmann, R. K., Killeen, S. Z., Maness, N. J., & Roy, C. J. (2021). Exhaled aerosol increases with COVID-19 infection, age, and obesity. *Proceedings of the National Academy of Sciences*, *118*(8), e2021830118. https://doi.org/10.1073/pnas.2021830118

Edwards, K. M., & Neuzil, K. M. (2022). Understanding COVID-19 through human challenge models. *Nature Medicine*, *28*(5), 903–904. https://doi.org/10.1038/s41591-022-01778-3

Egesa, M., Ssali, A., Tumwesige, E., Kizza, M., Driciru, E., Luboga, F., Roestenberg, M., Seeley, J., & Elliott, A. M. (2022). Ethical and practical considerations arising from community consultation on implementing controlled human infection studies using Schistosoma mansoni in Uganda. *Global Bioethics*, *33*(1), 78–102. https://doi.org/10.1080/11287462.2022.2091503

Eisinger, R. W. (2017). Email regarding consequences of misunderstanding about media coverage of report.

Ellenberg, S. S., & DeMets, D. L. (2016). Clinical trials series: Data monitoring committees-expect the unexpected. *New England Journal of Medicine*, *375*(14), 1365.

Ellis, H. (2021). James Phipps, first to be vaccinated against smallpox by Edward Jenner. *Journal of Perioperative Practice*, *31*(1-2), 51–52. https://doi.org/10.1177/1750458920950165

Emanuel, E. J. (2005). Undue inducement: Nonsense on stilts? *American Journal of Bioethics, 5*(5), 9–13. https://doi.org/10.1080/15265160500244959

Emanuel, E. J., Wendler, D., & Grady, C. (2000). What makes clinical research ethical? *Journal of the American Medical Association, 283*(20), 2701–2711. https://doi.org/10.1001/jama.283.20.2701

Emanuel, E. J., Wendler, D., Killen, J., & Grady, C. (2004). What Makes clinical research in developing countries ethical? The benchmarks of ethical research. *Journal of Infectious Diseases, 189*(5):930–937. https://doi.org/10.1086/381709

Eyal, N. (2020). The case to infect volunteers with COVID-19 to accelerate vaccine testing. TED Conference. Retrieved from https://www.ted.com/talks/nir_eyal_the_case_to_infect_volunteers_with_covid_19_to_accelerate_vaccine_testing

Eyal, N. (2024). Research ethics and public trust in vaccines: The case of COVID-19 challenge trials. *Journal of Medical Ethics, 50*(4), 278–284. https://doi.org/10.1136/medethics-2021-108086

Eyal, N., & Lipsitch, M. (2021). Testing SARS-CoV-2 vaccine efficacy through deliberate natural viral exposure. *Clinical Microbiology and Infection, 27*(3), 372–377. https://doi.org/https://doi.org/10.1016/j.cmi.2020.12.032

Eyal, N., Lipsitch, M., & Smith, P. G. (2020). Human challenge studies to accelerate coronavirus vaccine licensure. *Journal of Infectious Disease, 221*(11), 1752–1756. https://doi.org/10.1093/infdis/jiaa152

Faden, R. R., & Beauchamp, T. L. (1986). *A history and theory of informed consent.* Oxford University Press.

Feinberg, J. (1984). *The moral limits of the criminal law.* Oxford University Press.

Fernandez Lynch, H. (2020). The right to withdraw from controlled human infection studies: Justifications and avoidance. *Bioethics, 34*(8), 833–848. https://doi.org/10.1111/bioe.12704

Fisher, J. A., McManus, L., Cottingham, M. D., Kalbaugh, J. M., Wood, M. M., Monahan, T., & Walker, R. L. (2018). Healthy volunteers' perceptions of risk in US Phase I clinical trials: A mixed-methods study. *PLoS Med, 15*(11), e1002698. https://doi.org/10.1371/journal.pmed.1002698

Fisher, J. A., McManus, L., Kalbaugh, J. M., & Walker, R. L. (2021). Phase I trial compensation: How much do healthy volunteers actually earn from clinical trial enrollment? *Clinical Trials, 18*(4), 477–487. https://doi.org/10.1177/17407745211011069

Flanagan, J. (2021). The case for challenge trials. *Cato Unbound.* Retrieved from https://www.cato-unbound.org/2021/03/09/jessica-flanigan/case-challenge-trials/

Flory, J., & Emanuel, E. (2004). Interventions to improve research participants' understanding in informed consent for research: A systematic review. *Journal of the American Medical Association, 292*(13), 1593–1601. https://doi.org/10.1001/jama.292.13.1593

Gagnon, A., Miller, M. S., Hallman, S. A., Bourbeau, R., Herring, D. A., Earn, D. J., & Madrenas, J. (2013). Age-specific mortality during the 1918 influenza pandemic: Unravelling the mystery of high young adult mortality. *PloS One, 8*(8), e69586. https://doi.org/10.1371/journal.pone.0069586

Gale, J., & Bloomberg. (2021). The U.K. plans to infect young volunteers with COVID-19 to learn more about the virus. Fortune Magazine. Retrieved from https://fortune.com/2021/02/18/uk-infections-volunteers-human-challe nge-study/

Gan, L., Chen, Y., Tan, J., Wang, X., & Zhang, D. (2022). Does potential antibody-dependent enhancement occur during SARS-CoV-2 infection after natural infection or vaccination? A meta-analysis. *BMC Infectious Diseases, 22*(1), 1–742. https://doi.org/10.1186/s12879-022-07735-2

Geddawy, A., Ibrahim, Y. F., Elbahie, N. M., & Ibrahim, M. A. (2017). Direct acting anti-hepatitis C virus drugs: Clinical pharmacology and future direction. *Journal of Translational Internal Medicine, 5*(1), 8–17. https://doi.org/10.1515/jtim-2017-0007

Geulayov, G., Mansfield, K., Jindra, C., Hawton, K., & Fazel, M. (2022). Loneliness and self-harm in adolescents during the first national COVID-19 lockdown: Results from a survey of 10,000 secondary school pupils in England. *Current Psychology (New Brunswick, N.J.), 43*(15), 14063–14074. https://doi.org/10.1007/s12144-022-03651-5

Glaze, E. R., Roy, M. J., Dalrymple, L. W., & Lanning, L. L. (2015). A comparison of the pathogenesis of Marburg virus disease in humans and non-human primates and evaluation of the suitability of these animal models for predicting clinical efficacy under the "animal rule." *Comparative Medicine, 65*(3), 241–259.

Glim, M. (2021). That record-breaking sprint to create a COVID-19 vaccine. *NIH Catalyst, 29*(5). Retrieved from https://irp.nih.gov/catalyst/29/5/that-record-breaking-sprint-to-create-a-covid-19-vaccine

Goldby, S. (1971). Experiments at the Willowbrook State School. *Lancet, 1*(7702), 749. https://doi.org/10.1016/s0140-6736(71)92009-5

Gordon, S. B., Sichone, S., Chirwa, A. E., Hazenberg, P., Kafuko, Z., Ferreira, D. M., Flynn, J., Fortune, S., Balasingam, S., Biagini, G. A., McShane, H., Mwandumba, H. C., Jambo, K., Dedha, K., Raj Sharma, N., Robertson, B. D., Walker, N. F., Morton, B., & Group, TB Controlled Human Infection Model Development Group. (2023). Practical considerations for a TB controlled human infection model (TB-CHIM); the case for TB-CHIM in Africa, a systematic review of the literature and report of 2 workshop discussions in UK and Malawi. *Wellcome Open Res, 8*, 71. https://doi.org/10.12688/wellcomeopenres.18767.2

Govero, J., Esakky, P., Scheaffer, S. M., Fernandez, E., Drury, A., Platt, D. J., Gorman, M. J., Richner, J. M., Caine, E. A., Salazar, V., Moley, K. H., & Diamond, M. S. (2016). Zika virus infection damages the testes in mice. *Nature (London), 540*(7633), 438–442. https://doi.org/10.1038/nature20556

Grady, C., Cummings, S., Rowbotham, M., McConnell, M., Ashley, E., & Kang, G. (2017). Informed Consent. *New England Journal of Medicine, 376*, 856–867. https://doi.org/10.1056/NEJMra1603773

Grady, C., Shah, S., Miller, F., Danis, M., Nicolini, M., Ochoa, J., Taylor, H., Wendler, D., & Rid, A. (2020). So much at stake: Ethical tradeoffs in accelerating SARSCoV2 vaccine development. *Vaccine, 38*(41), 6381–6387. https://doi.org/https://doi.org/10.1016/j.vaccine.2020.08.017

Greenberg, J. S., Bruess, C. E., & Oswalt, S. B. (2013). Sexuality research. In J. S. Greenberg, C. E. Bruess, & S. B. Oswalt (Eds.), *Exploring the dimensions of human sexuality* (pp. 30–67). Jones & Bartlett Learning.

Grimwade, O., Savulescu, J., Giubilini, A., Oakley, J., & Nussberger, A.-M. (2020). Fair go: Pay research participants properly or not at all. *Journal of Medical Ethics, 46*, 837. https://doi.org/10.1136/medethics-2020-107060

Grimwade, O., Savulescu, J., Giubilini, A., Oakley, J., Osowicki, J., Pollard, A. J., & Nussberger, A. M. (2020). Payment in challenge studies: Ethics, attitudes and a new payment for risk model. *Journal of Medical Ethics, 46*(12), 815–826. https://doi.org/10.1136/medethics-2020-106438

Groome, M. J. D., Koen, A. M. D., Fix, A. M. D., Page, N. P., Jose, L. M. D., Madhi, S. A. P., McNeal, M. M. S., Dally, L. M., Cho, I. M. S., Power, M. M. P. H., Flores, J. M. D., & Cryz, S. P. (2017). Safety and immunogenicity of a parenteral P2-VP8-P[8] subunit rotavirus vaccine in toddlers and infants in South Africa: A randomised, double-blind, placebo-controlled trial. *Lancet Infectious Diseases, 17*(8), 843–853. https://doi.org/10.1016/S1473-3099(17)30242-6

Gupta, R. K., Abdul-Jawad, S., McCoy, L. E., Mok, H. P., Peppa, D., Salgado, M., Martinez-Picado, J., Nijhuis, M., Wensing, A. M. J., Lee, H., Grant, P., Nastouli, E., Lambert, J., Pace, M., Salasc, F., Monit, C., Innes, A. J., Muir, L., Waters, L., . . . Olavarria, E. (2019). HIV-1 remission following CCR5Delta32/Delta32 haematopoietic stem-cell transplantation. *Nature, 568*(7751), 244–248. https://doi.org/10.1038/s41586-019-1027-4

Gupta, S., Cohen, E., & Howard, J. (2020). US considering coronavirus strain for potential human challenge trials—but there's no intention to use it, Fauci says. *CNN.* https://www.cnn.com/2020/08/14/health/coronavirus-vaccine-strain-us-scientists-bn

Halpern, S. A. (2021). *Dangerous medicine: The story behind human experiments with hepatitis.* Yale University Press.

Halpern, S. D., Chowdhury, M., Bayes, B., Cooney, E., Hitsman, B. L., Schnoll, R. A., Lubitz, S. F., Reyes, C., Patel, M. S., Greysen, S. R., Mercede, A., Reale, C., Barg, F. K., Volpp, K. G., Karlawish, J., & Stephens-Shields, A. J. (2021). Effectiveness and ethics of incentives for research participation: 2 Randomized clinical trials. *JAMA Internal Medicine, 181*(11), 1479–1488. https://doi.org/10.1001/jamainternmed.2021.5450

Halstead, S. B. (2020). An urgent need for "common cold units" to study COVID-19. *American Journal of Tropical Medicine and Hygiene, 102*(6), 1152–1153. https://doi.org/10.4269/ajtmh.20-0246

Harbin, A., Laventhal, N., & Navin, M. (2023). Ethics of age de-escalation in pediatric vaccine trials: Attending to the case of COVID-19. *Vaccine, 41*(9), 1584–1588. https://doi.org/10.1016/j.vaccine.2023.01.055

Harrison, A. G., Lin, T., & Wang, P. (2020). Mechanisms of SARS-CoV-2 transmission and pathogenesis. *Trends in Immunology, 41*(12), 1100–1115. https://doi.org/10.1016/j.it.2020.10.004

Havervall, S., Ng, H., Jernbom Falk, A., Greilert-Norin, N., Månberg, A., Marking, U., Laurén, I., Gabrielsson, L., Salomonsson, A. C., Aguilera, K., Kihlgren, M., Månsson, M., Rosell, A., Hellström, C., Andersson, E., Olofsson, J., Skoglund, L., Yousef, J., Pin, E., . . . Thålin, C. (2022). Robust humoral and cellular immune responses and low risk for reinfection at least 8 months following asymptomatic to mild COVID-19. *Journal of Internal Medicine, 291*(1), 72–80. https://doi.org/10.1111/joim.13387

Henry, L. M., Larkin, M. E., & Pike, E. R. (2015). Just compensation: A no-fault proposal for research-related injuries. *Journal of Law and Bioscience*, 2(3), 645–668. https://doi.org/10.1093/jlb/lsv034

Herrera, S., Fernandez, O., Manzano, M. R., Murrain, B., Vergara, J., Blanco, P., Palacios, R., Velez, J. D., Epstein, J. E., Chen-Mok, M., Reed, Z. H., & Arevalo-Herrera, M. (2009). Successful sporozoite challenge model in human volunteers with Plasmodium vivax strain derived from human donors. *American Journal of Tropical Medicine and Hygiene*, 81(5), 740–746. https://doi.org/10.4269/ajtmh.2009.09-0194

Higgins-Dunn, N. L. B. (2020). Dr. Fauci says U.S. could return to normal by midfall if most people get Covid vaccine. *CNBC*. Retrieved from https://www.cnbc.com/2020/12/16/dr-fauci-says-us-could-return-to-normal-by-mid-fall-if-most-people-get-covid-vaccine.html

Hodgson, S. H., Juma, E., Salim, A., Magiri, C., Kimani, D., Njenga, D., Muia, A., Cole, A. O., Ogwang, C., Awuondo, K., Lowe, B., Munene, M., Billingsley, P. F., James, E. R., Gunasekera, A., Sim, B. K. L., Njuguna, P., Rampling, T. W., Richman, A., . . . Marsh, K. (2014). Evaluating controlled human malaria infection in Kenyan adults with varying degrees of prior exposure to Plasmodium falciparum using sporozoites administered by intramuscular injection. *Frontiers in Microbiology*, 5, 686. https://doi.org/10.3389/fmicb.2014.00686

Holm, S. (2020). Controlled human infection with SARS-CoV-2 to study COVID-19 vaccines and treatments: Bioethics in Utopia. *Journal of Medical Ethics*, 46(9), 569–573. https://doi.org/10.1136/medethics-2020-106476

Hoogerwerf, M. A., de Vries, M., & Roestenberg, M. (2020). Money-oriented risk-takers or deliberate decision-makers: A cross-sectional survey study of participants in controlled human infection trials. *BMJ Open*, 10(7), e033796. https://doi.org/10.1136/bmjopen-2019-033796

Hope, T., & McMillan, J. (2004). Challenge studies of human volunteers: Ethical issues. *Journal of Medical Ethics*, 30(1), 110–116. https://doi.org/10.1136/jme.2003.004440

Hou, Y., Zhao, S., Liu, Q., Zhang, X., Sha, T., Su, Y., Zhao, W., Bao, Y., Xue, Y., & Chen, H. (2022). Ongoing positive selection drives the evolution of SARS-CoV-2 genomes. *Genomics Proteomics Bioinformatics*, 20(6), 1214–1223. https://doi.org/10.1016/j.gpb.2022.05.009

Hsia, Y. E. (1999). Time changes all things, yet there is nothing new under the sun: The transience of ethical norms. *Politics and the Life Sciences*, 18(2), 312–314. https://doi.org/10.1017/S0730938400021560

Hughes, R. C. (2012). Individual risk and community benefit in international research. *Journal of Medical Ethics*, 38(10), 626–629. https://doi.org/10.1136/medethics-2011-100171

Hurst, S. A. (2008). Vulnerability in research and health care: Describing the elephant in the room? *Bioethics*, 22(4), 191–202. https://doi.org/10.1111/j.1467-8519.2008.00631.x

Hurst, S. A. (2014). Declaration of Helsinki and protection for vulnerable research participants. *Journal of the American Medical Association*, 311(12), 1252–1252. https://doi.org/10.1001/jama.2014.1272

Imperial College London. (2023). Participant information sheet. Imperial College Healthcare. Retrieved from https://www.imperial.ac.uk/media/imperial-coll ege/medicine/infectious-disease/COVHIC002_PIS_V5.0_17.10.2023.pdf

Indian Council of Medical Research. (2023a). ICMR consensus policy statement on the ethical conduct of controlled human infection studies (CHIS) in India (draft). Retrieved from https://main.icmr.nic.in/content/public-consultation-icmr-consensus-policy-statement-ethical-conduct-controlled-human

Indian Council of Medical Research. (2023b). Policy statement for the ethical conduct of controlled human infection studies (CHIS) in India. Retrieved from https://main.icmr.nic.in/sites/default/files/upload_documents/ICMR_C HIS%20_Policy_Document.pdf

Jackson, S., Marshall, J. L., Mawer, A., Lopez Ramon, R., Harris, S. A., Satti, I., Hughes, E., Preston-Jones, H., Cabrera Puig, I., Longet, S., Tipton, T., Laidlaw, S., Powell Doherty, R., Morrison, H., Mitchell, R., Ateere, A., Stylianou, E., Wu, M. S., Fredsgaard-Jones, T. P. W., . . . McShane, H. (2023). S109 A seropositive SARS-CoV-2 controlled human infection model demonstrating potent protective immunity and identification of immune correlates of protection. *Thorax*, *78*(Suppl 4), A78–A79. https://doi.org/10.1136/thorax-2023-BTSabstracts.115

Jackson, S., Marshall, J. L., Mawer, A., Lopez-Ramon, R., Harris, S. A., Satti, I., Hughes, E., Preston-Jones, H., Cabrera Puig, I., Longet, S., Tipton, T., Laidlaw, S., Doherty, R. P., Morrison, H., Mitchell, R., Tanner, R., Ateere, A., Stylianou, E., Wu, M.-S., . . . Vuddamalay, G. (2024). Safety, tolerability, viral kinetics, and immune correlates of protection in healthy, seropositive UK adults inoculated with SARS-CoV-2: A single-centre, open-label, phase 1 controlled human infection study. *The Lancet Microbe*, *5*(7), 655–668. https://doi.org/10.1016/ S2666-5247(24)00025-9

Jamrozik, E. (2018). How to hold an ethical pox party. *Journal of Medical Ethics*, *44*(4), 257–261. https://doi.org/10.1136/medethics-2017-104336

Jamrozik, E., Littler, K., Bull, S. Emerson, C., Kang, G., Kapulu, M., Rey, E., Saenz, C., Shah, S., Smith, P. G., Upshur, R., Weijer, C., & Selgelid, M. J. (2021). Key criteria for the ethical acceptability of COVID-19 human challenge studies: Report of a WHO Working Group. *Vaccine*, *39*(4), 633–640. https://doi.org/ 10.1016/j.vaccine.2020.10.075

Jamrozik, E., & Selgelid, M. J. (2020). COVID-19 human challenge studies: Ethical issues. *Lancet Infectious Disease*, *20*(8), e198–e203. https://doi.org/10.1016/ S1473-3099(20)30438-2

Jamrozik, E., & Selgelid, M. J. (2020). *Human challenge studies in endemic settings: Ethical and regulatory issues* (1st ed.). Springer Cham. https://doi.org/https:// doi.org/10.1007/978-3-030-41480-1

Jamrozik, E., & Selgelid, M. J. (2020b). Human infection challenge studies in endemic settings and/or low-income and middle-income countries: Key points of ethical consensus and controversy. *Journal of Medical Ethics*, *46*(9), 601–609. https://doi.org/10.1136/medethics-2019-106001

Jenner, E. (1802). An inquiry into the causes and effects of the variolae vaccinae disease discovered in some of the western counties of England, particularly Gloucestershire, and known by the name of the cow pox. Samuel, C. Retrieved from http://resource.nlm.nih.gov/2559001R

Joffe, S., Babiker, A., Ellenberg, S. S., Fix, A., Griffin, M. R., Hunsberger, S., Kalil, J., Levine, M. M., Makgoba, M. W., Moore, R. H., Tsiatis, A. A., & Whitley, R. (2021). Data and safety monitoring of COVID-19 vaccine clinical trials. *Journal of Infectious Diseases*, *224*(12), 1995–2000. https://doi.org/10.1093/infdis/jiab 263

Johnson, R. A., Rid, A., Emanuel, E., & Wendler, D. (2016). Risks of phase I research with healthy participants: A systematic review. *Clinical Trials*, *13*(2), 149–160. https://doi.org/10.1177/1740774515602868

Johnson, R. A., & Wendler, D. (2015). Challenging the sanctity of donorism: Patient tissue providers as payment-worthy contributors. *Kennedy Institute Ethics Journal*, *25*(3), 291–333. https://doi.org/10.1353/ken.2015.0021

Jongo, S., Church, L. W. P., Milando, F., Qassim, M., Schindler, T., Rashid, M., Tumbo, A., Nyaulingo, G., Bakari, B. M., Athuman Mbaga, T., Mohamed, L., Kassimu, K., Simon, B. S., Mpina, M., Zaidi, I., Duffy, P. E., Swanson, P. A., 2nd, Seder, R., Herman, J. D., . . . Hoffman, S. L. (2024). Safety and protective efficacy of PfSPZ vaccine administered to HIV-negative and -positive Tanzanian adults. *Journal of Clinical Investigation*, *134*(6), e169060. https://doi.org/10.1172/ JCI169060

Jongo, S. A., Shekalaghe, S. A., Church, L. W. P., Ruben, A. J., Schindler, T., Zenklusen, I., Rutishauser, T., Rothen, J., Tumbo, A., Mkindi, C., Mpina, M., Mtoro, A. T., Ishizuka, A. S., Kassim, K. R., Milando, F. A., Qassim, M., Juma, O. A., Mwakasungula, S., Simon, B., . . . Hoffman, S. L. (2018). Safety, immunogenicity, and protective efficacy against controlled human malaria infection of Plasmodium falciparum sporozoite vaccine in Tanzanian adults. *American Journal of Tropical Medicine and Hygiene*, *99*(2), 338–349. https://doi.org/ 10.4269/ajtmh.17-1014

Jurden A., Jacob, V. D., Long, K., Marsh, A., Eyal, N., Darton, T. C., Peeler, M., & Shah, S. K. (2024). Views of volunteers for SARS-CoV-2 CHI research.

Kahn, J. P., Henry, L. M., Mastroianni, A. C., Chen, W. H., & Macklin, R. (2020). Opinion: For now, it's unethical to use human challenge studies for SARS-CoV-2 vaccine development. *Proceedings of the National Academy of Science USA*, *117*(46), 28538–28542. https://doi.org/10.1073/pnas.2021189117

Kanazawa, J., Rawlings, S. A., Hendrickx, S., Gianella, S., Concha-Garcia, S., Taylor, J., Kaytes, A., Patel, H., Ndukwe, S., Little, S. J., Smith, D., & Dubé, K. (2023). Lessons learned from the Last Gift study: Ethical and practical challenges faced while conducting HIV cure-related research at the end of life. *Journal of Medical Ethics*, *49*(5), 305. https://doi.org/10.1136/medethics-2021-107512

Karron, R. (2019). Email sharing ethics consultation report from Johns Hopkins.

Kass, L. (1998). The wisdom of repugnance: Why we should ban the cloning of humans. *Valparaiso University Law Review*, *32*(2), 679–705.

Katzer, M., Salloch, S., Schindler, C., & Mertz, M. (2023). Ethical requirements for human challenge studies: A systematic review of reasons. *Clinical Pharmacology and Therapy*, *114*(6), 1209–1219. https://doi.org/10.1002/cpt.3054

Ke, R., Martinez, P. P., Smith, R. L., Gibson, L. L., Mirza, A., Conte, M., Gallagher, N., Luo, C. H., Jarrett, J., Zhou, R., Conte, A., Liu, T., Farjo, M., Walden, K. K. O., Rendon, G., Fields, C. J., Wang, L., Fredrickson, R., Edmonson, D. C., . . . Brooke, C. B. (2022). Daily longitudinal sampling of SARS-CoV-2 infection reveals substantial heterogeneity in infectiousness. *Nature Microbiology*, 7(5), 640–652. https://doi.org/10.1038/s41564-022-01105-z

Kelly, D. R. (2011). *Yuck!: The nature and moral significance of disgust*. MIT Press.

Kennedy, B., Tyson, A., & Funk, C. (2022). Americans' trust in scientists, other groups declines. *Pew Research Center*. Retrieved from https://www.pewresea rch.org/science/2022/02/15/americans-trust-in-scientists-other-groups-decli nes/

Kestelyn, E., Le Phuong, C., Ilo Van Nuil, J., Dong Thi, H. T., Minh Nguyen, N., Dinh The, T., Chambers, M., Simmons, C. P., Nguyen Trong, T., Nguyen The, D., Phuong, L. T., Do Van, D., Duc Anh, D., Nguyen Van, V. C., Baker, S., & Wills, B. (2019). Expert voices and equal partnerships: Establishing controlled human infection models (CHIMs) in Vietnam. *Wellcome Open Research*, 4, 143. https://doi.org/10.12688/wellcomeopenres.15337.1

Kettler, S. (2020). Fred Rogers took a stand against racial inequality when he invited a black character to join him in a pool. Biography. Retrieved from https://www.biography.com/actors/mister-rogers-officer-clemmons-pool

Khan, S., Akbar, S. M. F., Mahtab, M. A., Uddin, M. N., Rashid, M. M., Yahiro, T., Hashimoto, T., Kimitsuki, K., & Nishizono, A. (2024). Twenty-five years of Nipah outbreaks in Southeast Asia: A persistent threat to global health. *IJID Regions*, 13, 100434. https://doi.org/https://doi.org/10.1016/j.ijregi.2024.100 434

Kiernan, V. (1996). Measles trial broke consent rules. *New Scientist*, 150(2036), 8. https://www.ncbi.nlm.nih.gov/pubmed/11660241

Killingley, B., Mann, A. J., Kalinova, M., Boyers, A., Goonawardane, N., Zhou, J., Lindsell, K., Hare, S. S., Brown, J., Frise, R., Smith, E., Hopkins, C., Noulin, N., Londt, B., Wilkinson, T., Harden, S., McShane, H., Baillet, M., Gilbert, A., . . . Chiu, C. (2022). Safety, tolerability and viral kinetics during SARS-CoV-2 human challenge in young adults. *Nature Medicine*, 28(5), 1031–1041. https://doi.org/10.1038/s41591-022-01780-9

Koopman, J. P. R., Driciru, E., & Roestenberg, M. (2021). Controlled human infection models to evaluate schistosomiasis and hookworm vaccines: Where are we now? *Expert Review of Vaccines*, 20(11), 1369–1371. https://doi.org/10.1080/14760584.2021.1951244

Koopman, J. P. R., Houlder, E. L., Janse, J. J., Casacuberta-Partal, M., Lamers, O. A. C., Sijtsma, J. C., de Dood, C., Hilt, S. T., Ozir-Fazalalikhan, A., Kuiper, V. P., Roozen, G. V. T., de Bes-Roeleveld, L. M., Kruize, Y. C. M., Wammes, L. J., Smits, H. H., van Lieshout, L., van Dam, G. J., van Amerongen-Westra, I. M., Meij, P., . . . Roestenberg, M. (2023). Safety and infectivity of female cercariae in Schistosoma-naïve, healthy participants: A controlled human Schistosoma mansoni infection study. *EBioMedicine*, 97, 104832–104832. https://doi.org/10.1016/j.ebiom.2023.104832

Kraft, S. A., Duenas, D. M., Kublin, J. G., Shipman, K. J., Murphy, S. C., & Shah, S. K. (2018). Exploring ethical concerns about human challenge studies: A qualitative study of controlled human malaria infection study participants' motivations and attitudes. *Journal of Empirical Research on Human Research Ethics*, 14(1), 49–60. https://doi.org/10.1177/1556264618820219

Kraft, S. A., Rohrig, A., Williams, A., & Shah, S. K. (2023). Better recognition for research participants: What society should learn from Covid-19. *British Medical*

Journal (Online), *380*, e071178–e071178. https://doi.org/10.1136/bmj-2022-071178

Krugman, S. (1971). Experiments at the Willowbrook State School. *Lancet*, *1*(7706), 966–967. https://doi.org/10.1016/s0140-6736(71)91462-0

Krugman, S. (1986). The Willowbrook hepatitis studies revisited: Ethical aspects. *Reviews of Infectious Diseases*, *8*(1), 157–162. https://doi.org/10.1093/clinids/8.1.157

Kuiper, V. P., Rosendaal, F. R., Kamerling, I. M. C., Visser, L. G., & Roestenberg, M. (2021). Assessment of risks associated with severe acute respiratory syndrome coronavirus 2 experimental human infection studies. *Clinical Infectious Diseases*, *73*(5), e1228–e1234. https://doi.org/10.1093/cid/ciaa1784

Kuter, B. J., Offit, P. A., & Poland, G. A. (2021). The development of COVID-19 vaccines in the United States: Why and how so fast? *Vaccine*, *39*(18), 2491–2495. https://doi.org/10.1016/j.vaccine.2021.03.077

Kyei-Barffour, I., Addo, S. A., Aninagyei, E., Ghartey-Kwansah, G., & Acheampong, D. O. (2021). Sterilizing Immunity against COVID-19: Developing Helper T cells I and II activating vaccines is imperative. *Biomedical Pharmacotherapy*, *144*, 112282. https://doi.org/10.1016/j.biopha.2021.112282

Lamers, M. M., & Haagmans, B. L. (2022). SARS-CoV-2 pathogenesis. *Nature Reviews Microbiology*, *20*(5), 270–284. https://doi.org/10.1038/s41579-022-00713-0

Largent, E. A., & Fernandez Lynch, H. (2017). Paying research participants: Regulatory uncertainty, conceptual confusion, and a path forward. *Yale Journal Health, Policy, Law, and Ethics*, *17*(1), 61–141. https://www.ncbi.nlm.nih.gov/pubmed/29249912

Larkin, M. E. (2015). Acoustic separation and biomedical research: Lessons from Indian regulation of compensation for research injury. *Journal of Law and Medical Ethics*, *43*(1), 105–115. https://doi.org/10.1111/jlme.12199

Lederer, S. E. (2008). Walter Reed and the yellow fever experiments. In E. J. Emanuel, C. Grady, R. A. Crouch, R. K. Lie, F. G. Miller, & D. Wendler (Eds.), *The Oxford textbook of clinical research ethics* (pp. 9–17). Oxford University Press.

Lederer, S. E. (2014). The challenges of challenge experiments. *New England Journal of Medicine*, *371*(8), 695–697. https://doi.org/10.1056/NEJMp1408554

Leffingwell, A. (1899). Dr. Leffingwell on Sanarelli's yellow fever experiments. National Anti-Vivisection Society. Retrieved from https://d.lib.ncsu.edu/collections/catalog/mc00456-001-bx0002-049-001#?c=&m=&s=&cv=&xywh=1078%2C-770%2C2417%2C6436

Lenharo, M. (2023). Scientists deliberately gave women Zika – here's why. *Nature (London)*, *623*(7985), 18–18. https://doi.org/10.1038/d41586-023-03289-8

Levine, C. (1988). Has AIDS changed the ethics of human subjects research? *Law, Medicine & Health Care*, *16*(3–4), 167–173. https://doi.org/10.1111/j.1748-720X.1988.tb01942.x

Levine, M. M., Abdullah, S., Arabi, Y. M., Darko, D. M., Durbin, A. P., Estrada, V., Jamrozik, E., Kremsner, P. G., Lagos, R., Pitisuttithum, P., Plotkin, S. A., Sauerwein, R., Shi, S.-L., Sommerfelt, H., Subbarao, K., Treanor, J. J., Vrati, S., King, D., Balasingam, S., . . . Restrepo, A. M. H. (2020). Viewpoint of a WHO Advisory Group tasked to consider establishing a closely-monitored challenge model of coronavirus disease 2019 (COVID-19) in healthy volunteers. *Clinical Infectious Diseases, 72*(11), 2035–2041. https://doi.org/10.1093/cid/ciaa1290

London, A. J. (2012). A non-paternalistic model of research ethics and oversight: Assessing the benefits of prospective review. *Journal of Law, Medicine & Ethics, 40*(4), 930–944. https://doi.org/10.1111/j.1748-720X.2012.00722.x

London, A. J., & Kimmelman, J. (2019). Clinical trial portfolios: A critical oversight in human research ethics, drug regulation, and policy. *Hastings Center Report, 49*(4), 31–41. https://doi.org/10.1002/hast.1034

London, A. J., & Kimmelman, J. (2020). Against pandemic research exceptionalism. *Science (American Association for the Advancement of Science), 368*(6490), 476–477. https://doi.org/10.1126/science.abc1731

Lucido, C. (2020). Ethics and professionalism on the frontline: Controlled human infection trials in COVID-19 vaccine development: Ethical considerations. *South Dakota Medicine, 73*(10), 490–492.

Lyerly, A. D., Beigi, R., Bekker, L. G., Chi, B. H., Cohn, S. E., Diallo, D. D., Eron, J., Faden, R., Jaffe, E., Kashuba, A., Kasule, M., Krubiner, C., Little, M., Mfustso-Bengo, J., Mofenson, L., Mwapasa, V., Mworeko, L., Myer, L., Penazzato, M., . . . Wolf, L. (2021). Ending the evidence gap for pregnancy, HIV and co-infections: Ethics guidance from the PHASES project. *Journal of the International AIDS Society, 24*(12), e25846–n/a. https://doi.org/10.1002/jia2.25846

Lyerly, A. D., Little, M. O., & Faden, R. (2008). The second wave: Toward responsible inclusion of pregnant women in research. *International Journal of Feminist Approaches to Bioethics, 1*(2), 5–22. https://doi.org/10.3138/ijfab.1.2.5

Lynch, H. F., & Bateman-House, A. (2020). Facilitating both evidence and access: Improving FDA's accelerated approval and expanded access pathways. *Journal of Law, Medicine & Ethics, 48*(2), 365–372. https://doi.org/10.1177/1073110520935352

Lynch, H. F., Darton, T. C., Levy, J., McCormick, F., Ogbogu, U., Payne, R. O., Roth, A. E., Shah, A. J., Smiley, T., & Largent, E. A. (2021). Promoting ethical payment in human infection challenge studies. *American Journal of Bioethics, 21*(3), 11–31. https://doi.org/10.1080/15265161.2020.1854368

MacKay, D., Jecker, N. S., Pitisuttithum, P., & Saylor, K. W. (2020). Selecting participants fairly for controlled human infection studies. *Bioethics, 34*(8), 771–784. https://doi.org/10.1111/bioe.12778

Macklin, R. (2021). Double standards redux. *Indian Journal of Medical Ethics, VI*(2), 1–7. https://doi.org/10.20529/ijme.2021.021

Macklin, R., & Sherwin, S. (1975). Experimenting on human subjects: Philosophical perspectives. *Case West Reserve Law Review, 25*(3), 434–471. https://www.ncbi.nlm.nih.gov/pubmed/11661163

Mandava, A., Pace, C., Campbell, B., Emanuel, E., & Grady, C. (2012). The quality of informed consent: Mapping the landscape. A review of empirical data from developing and developed countries. *Journal of Medical Ethics, 38*(6), 356–365. https://doi.org/10.1136/medethics-2011-100178

Manson, P. (1900). Experimental proof of the mosquito malaria theory. *British Medical Journal, 2*(2074), 949–951. https://doi.org/10.1136/bmj.2.2074.949

Marsh, A. A., Magalhaes, M., Peeler, M., Rose, S. M., Darton, T. C., Eyal, N., Morrison, J., Shah, S. K., & Schmit, V. (2022). Characterizing altruistic motivation in potential volunteers for SARS-CoV-2 challenge trials. *PLoS One*, *17*(11), e0275823. https://doi.org/10.1371/journal.pone.0275823

Marsh, V. (2018). Exploring terminology and naming for controlled human infection models. Wellcome Trust. Retrieved from https://wellcome.org/sites/defa ult/files/exploring-terminology-and-naming-for-controlled-human-infection-models.pdf

Martinez-Perez, A., Ha, C., Whitehead, S., Durbin, A., & Weiskopf, D. (2024). Adaptive immune responses in a controlled human Zika challenge model. *Journal of Immunology*, *212*(1 Suppl), 0910_4482. https://doi.org/10.4049/jimmunol.212.supp.0910.4482

Matsui, K., Inoue, Y., & Yamamoto, K. (2021). SARS-CoV-2 human challenge trials: Rethinking the recruitment of healthy young adults first. *Ethics and Human Research*, *43*(3), 37–41. https://doi.org/10.1002/eahr.500089

McManus, L., Davis, A., Forcier, R. L., & Fisher, J. A. (2019). Appraising harm in Phase I trials: Healthy Volunteers' accounts of adverse events. *Journal of Law and Medical Ethics*, *47*(2), 323–333. https://doi.org/10.1177/1073110519857 289

McNeil Jr, D. G. (2017). They swallowed live typhoid bacteria – On purpose. *The New York Times*. Retrieved from https://www.nytimes.com/2017/09/28/hea lth/typhoid-vaccine-trial.html

McPartlin, S. O., Morrison, J., Rohrig, A., & Weijer, C. (2020). Covid-19 vaccines: Should we allow human challenge studies to infect healthy volunteers with SARS-CoV-2? *British Medical Journal*, *371*, m4258. https://doi.org/10.1136/bmj.m4258

Mehra, A. (2009). Politics of participation: Walter Reed's yellow-fever experiments. *Virtual Mentor*, *11*(4), 326–330. https://doi.org/10.1001/virtualmen tor.2009.11.4.mhst1-0904

Mello, M. M., Goodman, S. N., & Faden, R. R. (2012). Ethical considerations in studying drug safety: The Institute of Medicine report. *New England Journal of Medicine*, *367*(10), 959–964. https://doi.org/10.1056/NEJMhle1207160

Melo, A. S. d. O., Aguiar, R. S., Amorim, M. M. R., Arruda, M. B., Melo, F. d. O., Ribeiro, S. T. C., Batista, A. G. M., Ferreira, T., dos Santos, M. P., Sampaio, V. V., Moura, S. R. M., Rabello, L. P., Gonzaga, C. E., Malinger, G., Ximenes, R., de Oliveira-Szejnfeld, P. S., Tovar-Moll, F., Chimelli, L., Silveira, P. P., ... Tanuri, A. (2016). Congenital Zika virus infection: Beyond neonatal microcephaly. *JAMA Neurology*, *73*(12), 1407–1416. https://doi.org/10.1001/jamaneurol.2016.3720

Metzger, W. G., Ehni, H. J., Kremsner, P. G., & Mordmuller, B. G. (2019). Experimental infections in humans-historical and ethical reflections. *Tropical Medicine and International Health*, *24*(12), 1384–1390. https://doi.org/ 10.1111/tmi.13320

Miller, F. G. (2004). Research ethics and misguided moral intuition. *Journal of Law and Medical Ethics*, *32*(1), 111–116. https://doi.org/10.1111/j.1748-720x.2004. tb00455.x

Miller, F. G. (2013). The Stateville penitentiary malaria experiments: A case study in retrospective ethical assessment. *Perspectives in Biology and Medicine*, *56*(4), 548–567. https://doi.org/10.1353/pbm.2013.0035

Miller, F. G., & Grady, C. (2001). The ethical challenge of infection-inducing challenge experiments. *Clinical Infectious Disease*, *33*(7), 1028–1033. https://doi. org/10.1086/322664

Miller, F. G., & Joffe, S. (2009). Limits to research risks. *Journal Medical Ethics*, *35*(7), 445–449. https://doi.org/10.1136/jme.2008.026062

Miller, F. G., & Rosenstein, D. L. (1997). Psychiatric symptom-provoking studies: An ethical appraisal. *Biological Psychiatry*, *42*(5), 403–409. https://doi.org/10.1016/S0006-3223(97)00189-3

Miller, F. G., & Wertheimer, A. (2007). Facing up to paternalism in research ethics. *Hastings Center Report*, *37*(3), 24–34. https://doi.org/10.1353/hcr.2007.0044

Mintz, K., Jardas, E., Shah, S., Grady, C., Danis, M., & Wendler, D. (2021). Enrolling minors in COVID-19 vaccine trials. *Pediatrics (Evanston)*, *147*(3), 1. https://doi.org/10.1542/peds.2020-040717

Montgomery, R. A., Stern, J. M., Lonze, B. E., Tatapudi, V. S., Mangiola, M., Wu, M., Weldon, E., Lawson, N., Deterville, C., Dieter, R. A., Sullivan, B., Boulton, G., Parent, B., Piper, G., Sommer, P., Cawthon, S., Duggan, E., Ayares, D., Dandro, A., . . . Stewart, Z. A. (2022). Results of two cases of pig-to-human kidney xeno-transplantation. *New England Journal of Medicine*, *386*(20), 1889–1898. https://doi.org/10.1056/NEJMoa2120238

Morrison, J. (2021). Publish the protocol for the UK SARS-CoV-2 human challenge study now. *BMJ Blog*. Retrieved from https://blogs.bmj.com/bmj/2021/03/23/publish-the-protocol-for-the-uk-sars-cov-2-human-challenge-study-now/

Msemburi, W., Karlinsky, A., Knutson, V., Aleshin-Guendel, S., Chatterji, S., & Wakefield, J. (2023). The WHO estimates of excess mortality associated with the COVID-19 pandemic. *Nature*, *613*(7942), 130–137. https://doi.org/10.1038/s41586-022-05522-2

Mtunthama Toto, N., Gooding, K., Kapumba, B. M., Jambo, K., Rylance, J., Burr, S., Morton, B., Gordon, S. B., & Manda-Taylor, L. (2021). "At first, I was very afraid": A qualitative description of participants' views and experiences in the first Human Infection Study in Malawi. *Wellcome Open Research*, *6*, 89. https://doi.org/10.12688/wellcomeopenres.16587.2

Mulligan, M. J., Lyke, K. E., Kitchin, N., Absalon, J., Gurtman, A., Lockhart, S., Neuzil, K., Raabe, V., Bailey, R., Swanson, K. A., Li, P., Koury, K., Kalina, W., Cooper, D., Fontes-Garfias, C., Shi, P.-Y., Türeci, Ö., Tompkins, K. R., Walsh, E. E., . . . Jansen, K. U. (2020). Phase I/II study of COVID-19 RNA vaccine BNT162b1 in adults. *Nature*, *586*(7830), 589–593. https://doi.org/10.1038/s41586-020-2639-4

Mumba, N., Njuguna, P., Chi, P., Marsh, V., Awuor, E., Hamaluba, M., Mauncho, C., Mwalukore, S., Masha, J., Mwangoma, M., Kalama, B., Alphan, H., Wambua, J., Bejon, P., Kamuya, D., & Kapulu, M. C. (2022). Undertaking community engagement for a controlled human malaria infection study in Kenya: Approaches and lessons learnt. *Frontiers in Public Health*, *10*, 793913. https://doi.org/10.3389/fpubh.2022.793913

Murphy, H. (2018). They're hosting parasitic worms in their bodies to help treat a neglected disease. *The New York Times*. Retrieved from https://www.nytimes.com/2018/03/01/health/parasitic-worms-schistosomiasis-trial.html

Murphy, S. C., Duenas, D. M., Richie, T. L., & Shah, S. K. (2020). Reexamining the categorical exclusion of pediatric participants from controlled human infection trials. *Bioethics*, *34*(8), 785–796. https://doi.org/10.1111/bioe.12788

Najera, R. F. (2020). Black history month: Onesimus spreads wisdom that saves lives of Bostonians during a smallpox epidemic. *History of Vaccines*. Retrieved from https://historyofvaccines.org/blog/black-history-month-onesimus-spre ads-wisdom-that-saves-lives-of-bostonians-during-a-smallpox-epidemic-2

National Center for Health Statistics. (2024). Deaths by week and state: Provisional death counts for COVID-19. Centers for Disease Control. Retrieved from https://www.cdc.gov/nchs/nvss/vsrr/covid19/index.htm

Ndebele, P. M., Wassenaar, D., Munalula, E., & Masiye, F. (2012). Improving understanding of clinical trial procedures among low literacy populations: An intervention within a microbicide trial in Malawi. *BMC Medical Ethics, 13*(1), 29–29. https://doi.org/10.1186/1472-6939-13-29

Nedelman, M. (2020). Coronavirus vaccine trial administers first dose to participant. *CNN.* Retrieved from https://www.cnn.com/2020/03/17/health/coronavi rus-vaccine-first-dose-participant/index.html

Nelwan, M. L. (2019). Schistosomiasis: Life cycle, diagnosis, and control. *Current Therapeutic Research, 91,* 5–9. https://doi.org/10.1016/j.curtheres.2019.06.001

Njue, M., Njuguna, P., Kapulu, M. C., Sanga, G., Bejon, P., Marsh, V., Molyneux, S., & Kamuya, D. (2018). Ethical considerations in controlled human malaria infection studies in low resource settings: Experiences and perceptions of study participants in a malaria Challenge study in Kenya. *Wellcome Open Research, 3,* 39. https://doi.org/10.12688/wellcomeopenres.14439.1

Nuremberg Military Tribunals. (1949). *Trials of war criminals before the Nuremberg Military Tribunals under Control Council Law No. 10.* U.S. Government Printing Office

Nussbaum, M. C. (2004a). Danger to human dignity: The revival of disgust and shame in the law. *The Chronicle of Higher Education, 50*(48), B6–B9.

Nussbaum, M. C. (2004b). *Hiding from Humanity: Disgust, Shame, and the Law.* Princeton University Press. Retrieved from http://www.jstor.org/stable/j.ctt7s f7k.6

Office for Human Research Protections. (2010). Withdrawal of subjects from research guidance. Department of Health and Human Services. Retrieved from https://www.hhs.gov/ohrp/regulations-and-policy/guidance/guidance-on-wit hdrawal-of-subject/

Oguti, B., Gibani, M., Darlow, C., Waddington, C., Jin, C., Plested, E., Campbell, D., Jones, C., Darton, T., & Pollard, A. (2019). Factors influencing participation in controlled human infection models: A pooled analysis from six enteric fever studies [version 1; peer review: 3 approved with reservations]. *Wellcome Open Research, 4,* 153. https://doi.org/10.12688/wellcomeopenres.15469.1

Omer, S. B., Benjamin, R. M., Brewer, N. T., Buttenheim, A. M., Callaghan, T., Caplan, A., Carpiano, R. M., Clinton, C., DiResta, R., Elharake, J. A., Flowers, L. C., Galvani, A. P., Lakshmanan, R., Maldonado, Y. A., McFadden, S. M., Mello, M. M., Opel, D. J., Reiss, D. R., Salmon, D. A., . . . Hotez, P. J. (2021). Promoting COVID-19 vaccine acceptance: Recommendations from the Lancet Commission on Vaccine Refusal, Acceptance, and Demand in the USA. *Lancet, 398*(10317), 2186–2192. https://doi.org/10.1016/s0140-6736(21)02507-1

Oxford Vaccine Group. (2020). *About this study.* University of Oxford. Retrieved from https://trials.ovg.ox.ac.uk/trials/covhic002-About%20this%20study

Packard, R. M. (2016). *A history of global health: Interventions into the lives of other peoples.* Johns Hopkins University Press. https://doi.org/https://doi.org/ 10.56021/9781421420325

Packard, R. M. (2018). Learning to learn from global health history. *Bulletin of the World Health Organization, 96*(4), 231–232. https://doi.org/10.2471/blt.18.030 418

Palacios, R., & Shah, S. K. (2019). When could human challenge trials be deployed to combat emerging infectious diseases? Lessons from the case of a Zika virus human challenge trial. *Trials, 20*(Suppl 2), 702. https://doi.org/10.1186/s13 063-019-3843-0

Paquette, E. T., & Shah, S. K. (2020). Towards identifying an upper limit of risk: A persistent area of controversy in research ethics. *Perspectives in Biology and Medicine, 63*(2), 327–345. https://doi.org/10.1353/pbm.2020.0022

Parkash, V., Jones, G., Martin, N., Steigmann, M., Greensted, E., Kaye, P., Layton, A. M., & Lacey, C. J. (2021). Assessing public perception of a sand fly biting study on the pathway to a controlled human infection model for cutaneous leishmaniasis. *Research Involvement and Engagement, 7*(1), 33–33. https://doi.org/10.1186/s40900-021-00277-y

Pasteur, L. (1881). On the germ theory. *Science, 2*(62), 420–422. Retrieved from http://www.jstor.org.turing.library.northwestern.edu/stable/2900535

Patterson, K. D. (1992). Yellow fever epidemics and mortality in the United States, 1693–1905. *Social Science & Medicine, 34*(8), 855–865. https://doi.org/10.1016/0277-9536(92)90255-o

Paz-Bailey, G., Rosenberg, E. S., Doyle, K., Munoz-Jordan, J., Santiago, G. A., Klein, L., Perez-Padilla, J., Medina, F. A., Waterman, S. H., Adams, L. E., Lozier, M. J., Bertrán-Pasarell, J., Garcia Gubern, C., Alvarado, L. I., & Sharp, T. M. (2018). Persistence of Zika virus in body fluids: Final report. *New England Journal of Medicine, 379*(13), 1234–1243. https://doi.org/10.1056/NEJMoa1613108

Pierce, J. R. (2003). "In the interest of humanity and the cause of science": The yellow fever volunteers. *Military Medicine, 168*(11), 857–863. Retrieved from https://www.ncbi.nlm.nih.gov/pubmed/14680037

Piggin, M., Smith, E., Mankone, P., Ndegwa, L., Gbesemete, D., Pristera, P., Bahrami-Hessari, M., Johnson, H., Catchpole, A. P., Openshaw, P. J. M., Chiu, C., Read, R. C., Ward, H., & Barker, C. (2022). The role of public involvement in the design of the first SARS-CoV-2 human challenge study during an evolving pandemic. *Epidemics, 41*, 100626. https://doi.org/10.1016/j.epidem.2022.100626

Pike, E. R. (2012). Recovering from research: A no-fault proposal to compensate injured research participants. *American Journal of Law & Medicine, 38*(1), 7–62. https://doi.org/10.1177/009885881203800101

Pike, E. R. (2014). In need of remedy: US policy for compensating injured research participants. *Journal of Medical Ethics, 40*(3), 182–185. http://www.jstor.org.turing.library.northwestern.edu/stable/43282952

Platt, J. L., & Cascalho, M. (2022). The future of transplantation. *New England Journal of Medicine, 387*(1), 77–78. https://doi.org/10.1056/NEJMe2207105

Plotkin, S. A., & Caplan, A. (2020). Extraordinary diseases require extraordinary solutions. *Vaccine, 38*(24), 3987–3988. https://doi.org/10.1016/j.vaccine.2020.04.039

Plotkin, S. L., & Plotkin, S. A. (2018). 1 - A short history of vaccination. In S. A. Plotkin, W. A. Orenstein, P. A. Offit, & K. M. Edwards (Eds.), *Plotkin's vaccines*

(7th edition) (pp. 1–15.e18). Elsevier. https://doi.org/https://doi.org/10.1016/
B978-0-323-35761-6.00001-8

Poomkudy, J. T., & Shah, S. K. (2024). Virtue ethics and the unsettled ethical questions in controlled human infection studies. *Bioethics, 38*(8), 692–701. https://doi.org/10.1111/bioe.13326

Potter, A. R. (1993). Combating blinding trachoma. *BMJ, 307*(6898), 213–214. https://doi.org/10.1136/bmj.307.6898.213

Pratt, B. (2021). Sharing power in global health research: An ethical toolkit for designing priority-setting processes that meaningfully include communities. *International Journal of Equity in Health, 20*(1), 127. https://doi.org/10.1186/s12939-021-01453-y

Presidential Commission for the Study of Bioethical Issues. (2011). *"Ethically impossible" STD research in Guatemala from 1946 to 1948.* U.S. Government Printing Office.

Public Health Service Historian, History of Medicine Division, National Library of Medicine. (March 2024). *Smallpox: A great and terrible scourge.* Smallpox: Variolation. https://www.nlm.nih.gov/exhibition/smallpox/index.html.

Rainey, J. M., Jr., Aleem, A., Ortiz, A., Yeragani, V., Pohl, R., & Berchou, R. (1987). A laboratory procedure for the induction of flashbacks. *American Journal of Psychiatry, 144*(10), 1317–1319. https://doi.org/10.1176/ajp.144.10.1317

Rapeport, G., Smith, E., Gilbert, A., Catchpole, A., McShane, H., & Chiu, C. (2021). SARS-CoV-2 human challenge studies: Establishing the model during an evolving pandemic. *New England Journal of Medicine, 385*(11), 961–964. https://doi.org/10.1056/NEJMp2106970

Reed, W. (1902). Recent researches concerning the etiology, propagation, and prevention of yellow fever, by the United States Army Commission. *The Journal of Hygiene, 2*(2), 101–119. https://doi.org/10.1017/s0022172400001856

Reed, W., & Carroll, J. (1900). A comparative study of the biological characters and pathogenesis of Bacillus X (Sternberg), Bacillus icteroides (Sanarelli), and the hog-cholera bacillus (Salmon and Smith). *Journal of Experimental Medicine, 5*(3), 215–270. https://doi.org/10.1084/jem.5.3.215

Republic of Kenya Ministry of Health. (2022). *Guidelines for the conduct of clinical trials in Kenya.* https://web.pharmacyboardkenya.org/download/guidelines-for-the-conduct-of-clinical-trials-in-kenya/

Research & Development Blueprint Team. (2020). Feasibility, potential value and limitations of establishing a closely monitored challenge model of experimental COVID-19 infection and illness in healthy young adult volunteers. World Health Organization. Retrieved from https://www.who.int/publications/m/item/feasibility-potential-value-and-limitations-of-establishing-a-closely-monitored-challenge-model-of-experimental-covid-19-infection-and-illness-in-healthy-young-adult-volunteers

Richie, T. L. (2019). Workshop on ethical considerations for involving vulnerable populations in human challenge trials.

Rid, A., Feld, J. J., Liang, T. J., & Weijer, C. (2023). Ethics of controlled human infection studies with Hepatitis C virus. *Clinical Infectious Diseases, 77*(Suppl 3), S216–S223. https://doi.org/10.1093/cid/ciad382

Rid, A., & Roestenberg, M. (2020). Judging the social value of controlled human infection studies. *Bioethics, 34*(8), 749–763. https://doi.org/10.1111/bioe.12794

Riedel, S. (2005). Edward Jenner and the history of smallpox and vaccination. *Baylor University Medical Center Proceedings, 18*(1), 21–25. https://doi.org/ 10.1080/08998280.2005.11928028

Riggs, P. K., Chaillon, A., Jiarg, G., Letendre, S. L., Tang, Y., Taylor, J., Kaytes, A., Smith, D. M., Dubé, K., & Gianella, S. (2022). Lessons for understanding central nervous system HIV reservoirs from the Last Gift Program. *Current HIV/AIDS Reports, 19*(6), 566–579. https://doi.org/10.1007/s11904-022-00628-8

Robinson, W. M., & Unruh, B. T. (2008). The hepatitis experiments at the Willowbrook State School. In E. J. Emanuel, C. Grady, R. A. Crouch, R. K. Lie, F. G. Miller, & D. Wendler (Eds.), *The Oxford textbook of clinical research ethics* (pp. 80–85). Oxford University Press.

Roestenberg, M., Hoogerwerf, M.A., Ferreira, D. M., Mordmuller, B., & Yazdanbakhsh, M. (2018). Experimental infection of human volunteers. *Lancet Infectious Disease, 18*(10), e312–e322. https://doi.org/10.1016/S1473-3099(18)30177-4

Rose, A. (2018). The ethics of volunteer selection and compensation in Controlled Human Infection Models in India. *Indian Journal of Medical Ethics, 3*(4), 285–289. https://doi.org/10.20529/IJME.2018.084

Rossi, S. L., Ebel, G. D., Shan, C., Shi, P.-Y., & Vasilakis, N. (2018). Did Zika virus mutate to cause severe outbreaks? *Trends in Microbiology (Regular Ed.), 26*(10), 877–885. https://doi.org/10.1016/j.tim.2018.05.007

Rothman, D. J. (1991). *Strangers at the bedside: A history of how law and bioethics transformed medical decision making.* Basic Books.

Rozo, M., & Gronvall, G. K. (2015). The reemergent 1977 H1N1 strain and the gain-of-function debate. *mBio, 6*(4), e01013–e0101315. https://doi.org/ 10.1128/mBio.01013-15

Samuel, S. (2020). The UK is about to start deliberately infecting volunteers with Covid-19 to test vaccines. *Vox.* Retrieved from https://www.vox.com/future-perfect/2020/11/17/21540773/covid-19-vaccine-human-challenge-trial-ethics

Sanmukhani, J., & Tripathi, C. B. (2011). Ethics in clinical research: The Indian perspective. *Indian Journal of Pharmaceutical Sciences, 73*(2), 125–130. https:// doi.org/10.4103/0250-474x.91564

Schaefer, G. O., Tam, C. C., Savulescu, J., & Voo, T. C. (2020). COVID-19 vaccine development: Time to consider SARS-CoV-2 challenge studies? *Vaccine, 38*(33), 5085–5088. https://doi.org/10.1016/j.vaccine.2020.06.007

Schaefer, G. O., & Wertheimer, A. (2010). The right to withdraw from research. *Kennedy Institute Ethics Journal, 20*(4), 329–352. https://www.ncbi.nlm.nih. gov/pubmed/21338028

Schaich Borg, J., Lieberman, D., & Kiehl, K. A. (2008). Infection, incest, and iniquity: Investigating the neural correlates of disgust and morality. *Journal of Cognitive Neuroscience, 20*(9), 1529–1546. https://doi.org/10.1162/ jocn.2008.20109

Scharff, D. P., Mathews, K. J., Jackson, P., Hoffsuemmer, J., Martin, E., & Edwards, D. (2010). More than Tuskegee: Understanding mistrust about research participation. *Journal of Health Care for the Poor and Underserved, 21*(3), 879–897. https://doi.org/10.1353/hpu.0.0323

Schmidt, C. W. (2008). The yuck factor: When disgust meets discovery. *Environmental Health Perspectives, 116*(12), A524–A527. https://doi.org/DOI 10.1289/ehp.116-a524

Schrick, L., Tausch, S. H., Dabrowski, P. W., Damaso, C. R., Esparza, J., & Nitsche, A. (2017). An early American smallpox vaccine based on horsepox. *New England Journal of Medicine, 377*(15), 1491–1492. https://doi.org/10.1056/NEJMc1707600

Schultz, M. G., & Morens, D. M. (2009). Charles-Jules-Henri Nicolle. *Emerging Infectious Diseases, 15*(9), 1519–1522. https://doi.org/10.3201/eid1509.090891

Secretary's Advisory Committee on Human Research Protections. (2022). The protection of non-subjects from research harm. U.S. Department of Health and Human Services. Retrieved from https://www.hhs.gov/ohrp/sachrp-committee/recommendations/tab-c-the-protection-of-non-subjects-from-research-harm.html

Selgelid, M. J. (2016). Gain-of-function research: Ethical analysis. *Science and Engineering Ethics, 22*(4), 923–964. https://doi.org/10.1007/s11948-016-9810-1

Shah, S. K., Gross, M., & Nebeker, C. (2022). Optimizing ethics engagement in research: Learning from the ethical complexities of studying opioid use in pregnancy. *Journal of Law, Medicine & Ethics, 50*(2), 339–347. https://doi.org/10.1017/jme.2022.61

Shah, S. K., & Jamrozik, E. (2020). Do-it-yourself vaccines for COVID-19. *Scientific American.* Retrieved from https://www.scientificamerican.com/article/do-it-yourself-vaccines-for-covid-19/

Shah, S. K., Kimmelman J., Lyerly A. D., Lynch H. F., McCutcheon F., Miller F. G., Palacios R., Pardo-Villamizar C., & Zorrilla C. (2017). *Ethical considerations for zika virus human challenge trials.* National Institute of Allergy and Infectious Diseases. Retrieved from https://www.niaid.nih.gov/sites/default/files/EthicsZikaHumanChallengeStudiesReport2017.pdf

Shah, S., & Wendler, D. (2010). Interpretation of the subjects' condition requirement: A legal perspective. *Journal of Law, Medicine & Ethics, 38*(2), 365–373. https://doi.org/10.1111/j.1748-720X.2010.00495.x

Shah, S., Wolitz, R., & Emanuel, E. (2013). Refocusing the responsiveness requirement. *Bioethics, 27*(3), 151–159. https://doi.org/10.1111/j.1467-8519.2011.01903.x

Shah, S. K., Kimmelman, J., Lyerly, A. D., Lynch, H. F., Miller, F. G., Palacios, R., Pardo, C. A., & Zorrilla, C. (2018). Bystander risk, social value, and ethics of human research. *Science, 360*(6385), 158–159. https://doi.org/10.1126/science.aaq0917

Shah, S. K., London, A. J., Mofenson, L., Lavery, J. V., John-Stewart, G., Flynn, P., Theron, G., Bangdiwala, S. I., Moodley, D., Chinula, L., Fairlie, L., Sekoto, T., Kakhu, T. J., Violari, A., Dadabhai, S., McCarthy, K., & Fowler, M. G. (2021). Ethically designing research to inform multidimensional, rapidly evolving policy decisions: Lessons learned from the PROMISE HIV Perinatal Prevention Trial. *Clinical Trials (London, England), 18*(6), 681–689. https://doi.org/10.1177/17407745211045734

Shah, S. K., Miller, F. G., Darton, T. C., Duenas, D., Emerson, C., Lynch, H. F., Jamrozik, E., Jecker, N. S., Kamuya, D., Kapulu, M., Kimmelman, J., MacKay, D., Memoli, M. J., Murphy, S. C., Palacios, R., Richie, T. L., Roestenberg, M., Saxena, A., Saylor, K., ... Rid, A. (2020). Ethics of controlled human infection to address COVID-19. *Science, 368*(6493), 832–834. https://doi.org/10.1126/science.abc1076

Shah, S. K., Miller, F., & Fernandez Lynch, H. (2020). The role of community engagement in addressing bystander risks in research: The case of a Zika virus controlled human infection study. *Bioethics, 34*(9), 883–892. https://doi.org/10.1111/bioe.12806

Shan, C., Xia, H., Haller, S. L., Azar, S. R., Liu, Y., Liu, J., Muruato, A. E., Chen, R., Rossi, S. L., Wakamiya, M., Vasilakis, N., Pei, R., Fontes-Garfias, C. R., Singh, S. K., Xie, X., Weaver, S. C., & Shi, P.-Y. (2020). A Zika virus envelope mutation preceding the 2015 epidemic enhances virulence and fitness for transmission. *Proceedings of the National Academy of Sciences, 117*(33), 20190–20197. https://doi.org/10.1073/pnas.2005722117

Shankar, P. (2019). Zika virus infection. *RGUHS Journal of Medical Sciences, 9*(2), 53–56.

Shapira, T., Monreal, I. A., Dion, S. P., Buchholz, D. W., Imbiakha, B., Olmstead, A. D., Jager, M., Désilets, A., Gao, G., Martins, M., Vandal, T., Thompson, C. A. H., Chin, A., Rees, W. D., Steiner, T., Nabi, I. R., Marsault, E., Sahler, J., Diel, D. G., . . . Jean, F. (2022). A TMPRSS2 inhibitor acts as a pan-SARS-CoV-2 prophylactic and therapeutic. *Nature (London), 605*(7909), 340–348. https://doi.org/10.1038/s41586-022-04661-w

Sharma, A., Apte, A., Rajappa, M., Vaz, M., Vaswani, V., Goenka, S., Malhotra, S., Sangoram, R., Lakshminarayanan, S., Jayaram, S., Mathaiyan, J., Farseena, K., Mukerjee, P., Jaswal, S., Dongre, A., Timms, O., Shafiq, N., Aggarwal, R., Kaur, M., . . . Kang, G. (2022). Perceptions about controlled human infection model (CHIM) studies among members of ethics committees of Indian medical institutions: A qualitative exploration. *Wellcome Open Research, 7*, 209. https://doi.org/10.12688/wellcomeopenres.17968.2

Sheehy, S. H., Douglas, A. D. & Draper, S. J. (2013). Challenges of assessing the clinical efficacy of asexual blood-stage Plasmodium falciparum malaria vaccines. *Human Vaccine and Immunotherapy, 9*(9), 1831–1840. https://doi.org/10.4161/hv.25383

Shekalaghe, S., Rutaihwa, M., Billingsley, P. F., Chemba, M., Daubenberger, C. A., James, E. R., Mpina, M., Ali Juma, O., Schindler, T., Huber, E., Gunasekera, A., Manoj, A., Simon, B., Saverino, E., Church, L. W. P., Hermsen, C. C., Sauerwein, R. W., Plowe, C., Venkatesan, M., . . . Hoffman, S. L. (2014). Controlled human malaria infection of Tanzanians by intradermal injection of aseptic, purified, cryopreserved Plasmodium falciparum sporozoites. *American Journal of Tropical Medicine and Hygiene, 91*(3), 471–480. https://doi.org/10.4269/ajtmh.14-0119

Simpson, D. I. H. (1964). Zika virus infection in man. *Transactions of the Royal Society of Tropical Medicine and Hygiene, 58*(4), 335–337. https://doi.org/10.1016/0035-9203(64)90201-9

Slaoui, M., & Hepburn, M. (2020). Developing safe and effective covid vaccines: Operation Warp Speed's strategy and approach. *New England Journal of Medicine, 383*(18), 1701–1703. https://doi.org/10.1056/NEJMp2027405

Smith, K. N. (2019). The young soldiers who fought yellow fever and won. Forbes. Retrieved from https://www.forbes.com/sites/kionasmith/2019/08/31/the-young-soldiers-who-fought-yellow-fever-and-won/?sh=97c852b67356

Smith, P. C. (2012). Reflections in the water society and recreational facilities, a case study of public swimming pools in Mississippi. *Southeastern Geographer, 52*(1), 39–54. https://doi.org/10.1353/sgo.2012.0000

Spence, S. E. W. (2020). COVID-19 vaccine trial reports high effectiveness; Umass Medical School key enrollment site. Retrieved from https://www.umassmed. edu/news/news-archives/2020/11/covid-19-vaccine-trial-reports-high-effect iveness-umass-medica-school-key-enrollment-site/

Spinola, S. M., Broderick, C., Zimet, G. D., & Ott, M. A. (2021). Human challenge studies with wild-type severe acute respiratory sydrome coronavirus 2 violate longstanding codes of human subjects research. *Open Forum Infectious Diseases, 8*(1), ofaa615–ofaa615. https://doi.org/10.1093/ofid/ofaa615

Stanisic, D. I., McCarthy, J. S., & Good, M. F. (2018). Controlled human malaria infection: Applications, advances, and challenges. *Infection and Immunity, 86*(1), e00479–e00496. https://doi.org/10.1128/iai.00479-17

Staples, J. E., & Monath, T. P. (2008). Yellow fever: 100 years of discovery. *Journal of the American Medical Association, 300*(8), 960–962. https://doi.org/10.1001/jama.300.8.960

Steel, R. (2020). Reconceptualising risk-benefit analyses: The case of HIV cure research. *Journal of Medical Ethics, 46*(3), 212–219. https://doi.org/10.1136/medethics-2019-105548

Sternberg, G. M. (1898). The bacillus icteroides (Sanarelli) and bacillus X (Sternberg). *Transactions of the Association of American Physicians, 13*, 71.

Strohminger, N. (2014a). Disgust talked about. *Philosophy Compass, 9*(7), 478–493. https://doi.org/https://doi.org/10.1111/phc3.12137

Strohminger, N. (2014b). The meaning of disgust: A refutation. *Emotion Review, 6*(3), 214–216. https://doi.org/10.1177/1754073914523072

Stunkel, L., & Grady, C. (2011). More than the money: A review of the literature examining healthy volunteer motivations. *Contemporary Clinical Trials, 32*(3), 342–352. https://doi.org/https://doi.org/10.1016/j.cct.2010.12.003

Su, S., Shao, Y., & Jiang, S. (2021). Human challenge trials to assess the efficacy of currently approved COVID-19 vaccines against SARS-CoV-2 variants. *Emerging Microbes and Infections, 10*(1), 439–441. https://doi.org/10.1080/22221751.2021.1896956

Sutter, P. S. (2016). "The first mountain to be removed": Yellow fever control and the construction of the Panama Canal. *Environmental History Durham North Carolina, 21*(2), 250–259.

Szczęśniak, M., & Brydak-Godowska, J. (2021). SARS-CoV-2 and the eyes: A review of the literature on transmission, detection, and ocular manifestations. *Medical Science Monitor, 27*, e931863–e931863. https://doi.org/10.12659/MSM.931863

Tavaglione, N., Martin, A. K., Mezger, N., Durieux-Paillard, S., François, A., Jackson, Y., & Hurst, S. A. (2015). Fleshing out vulnerability. *Bioethics, 29*(2), 98–107. https://doi.org/10.1111/bioe.12065

Theodosiou, A. A., Laver, J. R., Dale, A. P., Cleary, D. W., Jones, C. E., & Read, R. C. (2022). Controlled human infection with Neisseria lactamica in late pregnancy to measure horizontal transmission and microbiome changes in mother–neonate pairs: A single-arm interventional pilot study protocol. *BMJ Open, 12*(5), e056081–e056081. https://doi.org/10.1136/bmjopen-2021-056081

Tomes, N. J. (1997). American attitudes toward the germ theory of disease: Phyllis Allen Richmond revisited. *Journal of the History of Medicine and Allied Sciences, 52*(1), 17–50. http://www.jstor.org.turing.library.northwestern.edu/stable/24624203

Trender, W., Hellyer, P. J., Killingley, B,. Kalinova, M., Mann, A. J., Catchpole, A. P., Menon, D., Needham, E., Thwaites, R., Chiu, C., Scott, G., & Hampshire, A. (2024). Changes in memory and cognition during the SARS-CoV-2 human challenge study. *eClincal Medicine, 76*(102842). https://www.thelancet.com/journals/eclinm/article/PIIS2589-5370(24)00421-8/fulltext

Tsuchiya, T. (2008). The Imperial Japanese experiments in China. In E. J. Emanuel, C. Grady, R. A. Crouch, R. K. Lie, F. G. Miller, & D. Wendler (Eds.), *The Oxford textbook of clinical research ethics* (pp. 31–45). Oxford University Press.

Tyrrell, D. A. (1992). A view from the Common Cold Unit. *Antiviral Research, 18*(2), 105–125. https://doi.org/10.1016/0166-3542(92)90032-z

U.S. Department of Health and Human Services. (1979). *Protection of human subjects; Belmont Report: Notice of report for public comment.* (pp. 0097–6326). Department of Health, Education, and Welfare.

van der Worp, H. B., Howells, D. W., Sena, E. S., Porritt, M. J., Rewell, S., O'Collins, V., & Macleod, M. R. (2010). Can animal models of disease reliably inform human studies? *PLOS Medicine, 7*(3), e1000245. https://doi.org/10.1371/journal.pmed.1000245

Vannice, K. S., Cassetti, M. C., Eisinger, R. W., Hombach, J., Knezevic, I., Marston, H. D., Wilder-Smith, A., Cavaleri, M., & Krause, P. R. (2019). Demonstrating vaccine effectiveness during a waning epidemic: A WHO/NIH meeting report on approaches to development and licensure of Zika vaccine candidates. *Vaccine, 37*(6), 863–868. https://doi.org/10.1016/j.vaccine.2018.12.040

Vaswani, V., Saxena, A., Shah, S. K., Palacios, R., & Rid, A. (2020). Informed consent for controlled human infection studies in low- and middle-income countries: Ethical challenges and proposed solutions. *Bioethics, 34*(8), 809–818. https://doi.org/10.1111/bice.12795

Vaz, M., Timms, O., Johnson, A. R., S, R. K., Ramanathan, M., & Vaz, M. (2021). Public perceptions on controlled human infection model (CHIM) studies: A qualitative pilot study from South India. *Monash Bioethics Review, 39*(1), 68–93. https://doi.org/10.1007/s40592-020-00121-1

Vaz, M., Timms, O., Rose, A., Manesh, A., & Bhan, A. (2019). Consultation on the feasibility and ethics of specific, probable Controlled Human Infection Model study scenarios in India: A report. *Indian Journal of Medical Ethics, 4*(3), 238–242.

Walker, R. L., & Fisher, J. A. (2019). "My body is one of the best commodities": Exploring the ethics of commodification in Phase I healthy volunteer clinical trials. *Kennedy Institute Ethics Journal, 29*(4), 305–331. https://doi.org/10.1353/ken.2019.0028

Walker, R. L., MacKay, D., Waltz, M., Lyerly, A. D., & Fisher, J. A. (2022). Ethical criteria for improved human subject protections in Phase I healthy volunteer trials. *Ethics in Human Research, 44*(5), 2–21. https://doi.org/10.1002/eahr.500139

Warner, M. (1985). Hunting the yellow fever germ: The principle and practice of etiological proof in late nineteenth-century America. *Bulletin of the History of Medicine, 59*(3), 361–382. Retrieved from https://www.ncbi.nlm.nih.gov/pubmed/3899228

Weijer, C. (2024). COVID-19 human challenge trials and randomized controlled trials: Lessons for the next pandemic. *Research Ethics, 20*(4), 17470161231223594. https://doi.org/10.1177/17470161231223594

Weindling, P. J. (2008). The Nazi medical experiments. In E. J. Emanuel, C. Grady, R. A. Crouch, R. K. Lie, F. G. Miller, & D. Wendler (Eds.), *The Oxford textbook of clinical research ethics* (pp. 18–30). Oxford University Press.

Wendler, D. (2010). *The ethics of pediatric research.* Oxford University Press.

Wendler, D., & Rid, A. (2017). In defense of a social value requirement for clinical research. *Bioethics, 31*(2), 77–86. https://doi.org/10.1111/bioe.12325

Wendler, D., & Varma, S. (2006). Minimal risk in pediatric research. *Journal of Pediatrics, 149*(6), 855–861. https://doi.org/10.1016/j.jpeds.2006.08.064

Wenner, D. M. (2017). The social value of knowledge and the responsiveness requirement for international research. *Bioethics, 31*(2), 97–104. https://doi.org/ 10.1111/bioe.12316

Wertheimer, A., & Miller, F. G. (2008). Payment for research participation: A coercive offer? *Journal of Medical Ethics, 34*(5), 389–392. https://doi.org/10.1136/ jme.2007.021857

Wertheimer, A., & Miller, F. G. (2014). There are (STILL) no coercive offers. *Journal of Medical Ethics, 40*(9), 592–593. https://doi.org/10.1136/medethics-2013-101510

Whitehead, C. L., & Walker, S. P. (2020). Consider pregnancy in COVID-19 therapeutic drug and vaccine trials. *Lancet (British edition), 395*(10237), e92. https:// doi.org/10.1016/S0140-6736(20)31029-1

WHO Working Group for Guidance on Human Challenge Studies in COVID-19. (2020). Key criteria for the ethical acceptability of COVID-19 human challenge studies. World Health Organization. Retrieved from https://www.who.int/publi cations/i/item/WHO-2019-nCoV-Ethics_criteria-2020.1

Wicclair, M. R. (2008). Ethics and research with deceased patients. *Cambridge Quarterly of Healthcare Ethics, 17*(1), 87–97. https://doi.org/10.1017/S09631 80108080092

Williams, E., Craig, K., Chiu, C., Davies, H., Ellis, S., Emerson, C., Jamrozik, E., Jefford, M., Kang, G., Kapulu, M., Kolstoe, S. E., Littler, K., Lockett, A., Elena, R., Messer, J., McShane, H., Saenz, C., Selgelid, M. J., Shah, S., . . . Yamazaki, N. (2022). Ethics review of COVID-19 human challenge studies: A joint HRA/ WHO workshop. *Vaccine, 40*(26), 3484–3489. https://doi.org/10.1016/j.vacc ine.2022.02.004

Williams, T. B., Badariotti, J. I., Corbett, J., Miller-Dicks, M., Neupert, E., McMorris, T., Ando, S., Parker, M. O., Thelwell, R. C., Causer, A. J., Young, J. S., Mayes, H. S., White, D. K., de Carvalho, F. A., Tipton, M. J., & Costello, J. T. (2024). The effects of sleep deprivation, acute hypoxia, and exercise on cognitive performance: A multi-experiment combined stressors study. *Physiology and Behavior, 274*, 114409. https://doi.org/10.1016/j.physbeh.2023.114409

World Health Organization's Council for International Organizations of Medical Sciences. (2016). *International ethical guidelines for health-related research involving humans.* World Health Organization. Retrieved from https://cioms. ch/wp-content/uploads/2017/01/WEB-CIOMS-EthicalGuidelines.pdf

World Health Organization. (WHO). (2022). *WHO guidance on the ethical conduct of controlled human infection studies.* Retrieved from https://www.who.int/publications/i/item/9789240037816

World Health Organization (WHO). (2024). Online public consultation on the draft key criteria for the ethical acceptability of controlled human infection studies during public health emergencies. Retrieved from https://www.who.int/news-room/articles-detail/online-public-consultation-on-the-draft-key-criteria-for-the-ethical-acceptability-of-controlled-human-infection-studies-during-public-health-emergencies

World Health Organization (WHO) (2020). *Ending the neglect to attain the Sustainable Development Goals: a road map for neglected tropical diseases 2021–2030.* World Health Organization. Licence: CC BY-NC-SA 3.0 IGO. Retrieved from https://www.who.int/publications/i/item/9789240010352

World Medical Association. (2013). Declaration of Helsinki: Ethical principles for medical research involving human subjects. *Journal of the American Medical Association, 310*(20), 2191–2194. https://doi.org/10.1001/jama.2013.281053

Yeragani, V. K., Balon, R., Rainey, J. M., Ortiz, A., Berchou, R., Lycaki, H., & Pohl, R. (1988). Effects of laboratory-induced panic-anxiety on subsequent provocative infusions. *Psychiatry Research, 23*(2), 161–166. https://doi.org/10.1016/0165-1781(88)90006-6

Yu, I. T. S., Li, Y., Wong, T. W., Tam, W., Chan, A. T., Lee, J. H. W., Leung, D. Y. C., & Ho, T. (2004). Evidence of airborne transmission of the severe acute respiratory syndrome virus. *New England Journal of Medicine, 350*(17), 1731–1739. https://doi.org/10.1056/NEJMoa032867

Yu, M., Darton, T. C., & Kimmelman, J. (2020). Decision analysis approach to risk/benefit evaluation in the ethical review of controlled human infection studies. *Bioethics, 34*(8), 764–770. https://doi.org/10.1111/bioe.12773

Zeng, W., Wang, X., Li, J., Yang, Y., Qiu, X., Song, P., Xu, J., & Wei, Y. (2020). Association of daily wear of eyeglasses with susceptibility to coronavirus disease 2019 infection. *JAMA Ophthalmology, 138*(11), 1196–1199. https://doi.org/10.1001/jamaophthalmol.2020.3906

Zhou, J., Singanayagam, A., Goonawardane, N., Moshe, M., Sweeney, F. P., Sukhova, K., Killingley, B., Kalinova, M., Mann, A. J., Catchpole, A. P., Barer, M. R., Ferguson, N. M., Chiu, C., & Barclay, W. S. (2023). Viral emissions into the air and environment after SARS-CoV-2 human challenge: A phase 1, open label, first-in-human study. *Lancet Microbe, 4*(8), e579–e590. https://doi.org/10.1016/S2666-5247(23)00101-5

Index